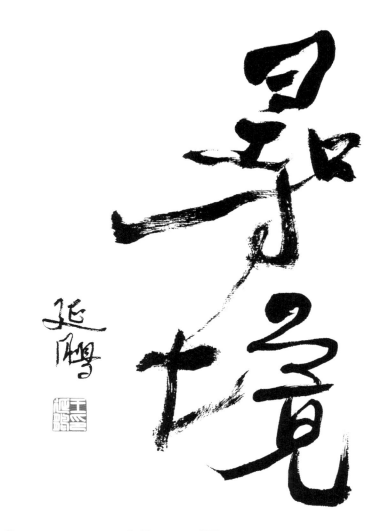

SEEKING NEW TERRITORY

生命之美显微摄影艺术

BEAUTY OF LIFE PHOTOMICROGRAPHY

李铁军 著

BY LI TIEJUN

人民卫生出版社
·北 京·

目录
CONTENTS

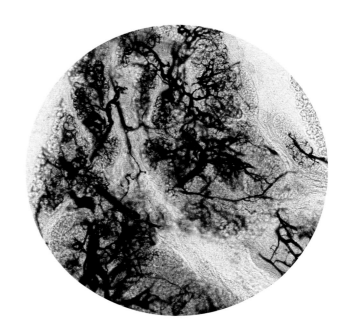
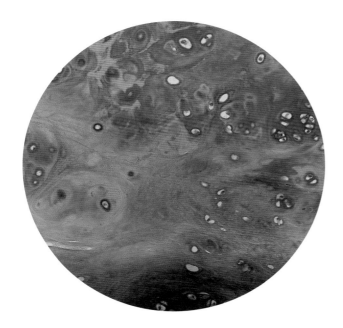

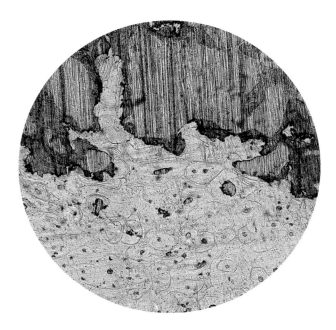

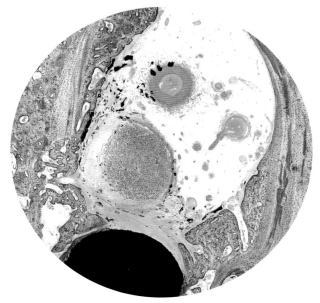

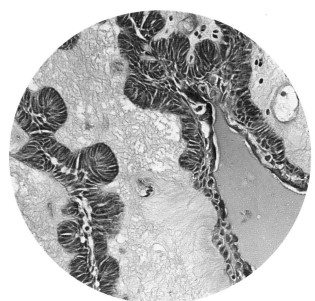

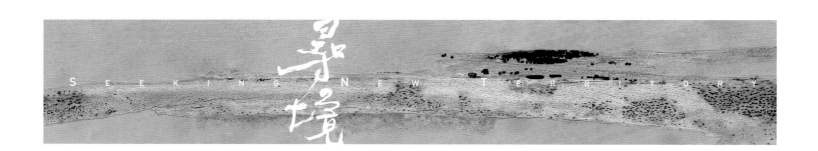

序言·寻境

彭志翔

中山大学光华口腔医学院教授

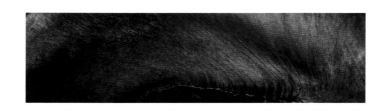

每一个生命都在跋涉中寻找。有的就找到了什么，比如李铁军先生，这位北大口腔病理学知名教授，在显微镜下的生命微观视野里，发现了另一方天地洪荒，它的包罗万象，与我们置身其中的宏观宇宙相比，完全不遑多让。那些景观令我们每个人惊叹不已。

其实在很久以前，智慧的光就已先于显微镜光束，同时照射进了宏观与微观世界。庄子就说过：天下莫大于秋豪之末，而太山为小。又说：天地与我并生，而万物与我为一。

所以，当我们将自己的身体放大之后，发现里面竟然有日月星辰、山岳海洋、鱼虫鸟兽、神话史诗等等一切时，就没有什么好奇怪的了。

李铁军教授以医学专家之身，跨界摄影，在科学与艺术之间作逍遥游，这提醒了我们重新去打量两者之间的关系。从器物角度观之，科学进步无疑助力了艺术的发展。十七世纪荷兰画家维米尔，就是因为与精通显微镜的科学家列文虎克交友，才能使用当时罕见的暗箱技术，捕捉光线和色彩，所以他的那些不朽名画，就有了一种非常明净和真实的影像光感；而从精神角度观之，那些登临或接近科学之巅的人们，一定也看到了艺术之光。如同爱因斯坦在那个历史性的早晨，突然魂不守舍时，走到钢琴前开始弹奏起来，就在一阵阵激荡的琴声中，相对论诞生了。

因此，科学与艺术，在至高的创造之境之中，是双向突破，

彼此相通的，一如米开朗基罗的壁画，《创世纪》中，上帝与亚当各自伸出的手，两个指尖眼看就要触碰到了，创造即将发生。那么，究竟是谁创造了谁，也许是一个言人人殊的问题。或者，他们彼此创造了对方。倘如此，人性与神性，就共存于你我体内了，如孟子曰："万物皆备于我矣"。当人类通过天文望远镜，窥探到浩瀚宇宙中，超新星的绚烂爆发时，有人会认为那是神对我们渺小人类投来的一瞥；而当我们打开显微镜，去探寻生命世界的微观景象时，那会不会就是，神把眼睛借给我们，让我们在上帝视角中去发现宇宙万物的奥秘？

西方哲学家有言：生命不过是一种想象，这种想象可以突破人世间的任何阻隔。当你看到李铁军教授对生命世界的一个个微观呈现，其中的意象之境有：大漠秋风、杏花江南、鱼翔浅底、鸥掠浪尖、明月冰川、落霞孤鹜、古墓残画、雪山豹骸，你就会发现，一个医学家在追寻真与美之境的路上前行着的身影。就像研究人体解剖的达·芬奇，期待去发现人体中蕴藏的，那个与大宇宙运行规则相同的小宇宙一样。这些人独具慧眼的追寻，最终都提升了我们。

也许，寻找的意义往往不在于止境之所得。山一程，水一程，你在跋涉中就一点点完成了自我修炼。愿我们每个人都在寻找美与真的路上，实现人的高贵与尊严。

PREFACE · SEEKING NEW TERRITORY

Peng Zhixiang

Professor, Guanghua School of Stomatology, Sun Yat-Sen University

Every life is a long journey of pursuit and search. Someone, like Mr. Li Tiejun, did find some enlightenments in his own journey of pursuing. In the microscopic view of life under his microscope, Mr. Li Tiejun, a well-known professor of oral pathology at Peking University, has discovered a rare-traveled territory — a mysterious and all-embracing micro-world that is absolutely comparable with the macro universe we are living in. These microscopic scenes of life have amazed us all.

In fact, long before the microscopic beam, light of wisdom had shined both onto the macro and micro worlds. Zhuang Zi once said that all in all, there is nothing bigger than the tip of rabbit's hair, and nothing smaller than the Mount Tai. He also believed that we are born with the heaven and the earth, thus everything in the universe, including us humans, is harmonized as one.

Therefore, there is no wonder that when we zoom in on our own body and find out that there are such things as sun, moon and stars, mountains and oceans, fish, birds and beasts, even mythological epics, and so on.

Professor Li Tiejun, a medical expert and a micrographic artist, enjoys his cross-border journey between science and art. This reminds us to re-examine the relationship between the two. From the perspective of artifacts, scientific progress has undoubtedly contributed to the renovation of art. In the seventeenth century, a Dutch painter Vermeer, as a friend of a famous scientist Leeuwenhoek who is proficient in the microscope, can use a rare kind of black box technique at that time to capture the light and color, so his immortal paintings have a very unique sense of lighting in the images. From a spiritual point of view, those who board or approach the top of science must have also seen the light of art. In that historic morning, as Albert Einstein suddenly stopped walking and rushed to the piano and began to play it. In the bursting sound of the piano, the famous theory of relativity was born.

Therefore, science and art, in the highest creative moments, are mutually two-way breakthroughs, which are interpenetrated to each other. Like in Michelangelo's famous mural painting—Genesis, God and Adam both extended their hands with fingertips. Seeing it is touching each other, the creation is about

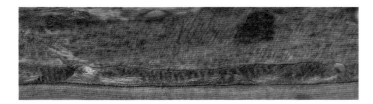 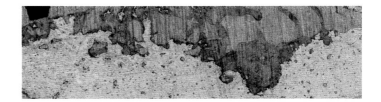

to happen. Then, one may ask who created whom? It is perhaps a question of disagreement. Or perhaps they created each other. If so, humanity and divinity may coexist in you and me, as Mencius said that everything in the world is harmonized in me. When human peek into the vast universe through astronomical telescopes and find the supernova's glorious outburst, some people may think that it is just a glimpse of God's look toward human beings; and when we explore the microscopic scene of life under the microscope, then it may well be that, God lends us his eyes, to let us discover the mysteries of the universe where God reveals himself.

Once a western philosopher said that life is merely just an imagination. It can break through any barrier in the world. When you see Professor Li Tiejun's micro-images of the world's lives, the beauty breaks free from the frames and knows no limits and assumes abundant shapes. Desert autumn wind, southern apricot flower, fish shoal in shallow water, gulls skimming the sea wave, glaciers under moon light, lonely crane flying in sunset, ancient tombs paintings, snow mountain leopard, and so on. Through these scenes, you may imagine a medical scientist

is stalking on the road of pursuing the true and beautiful world, just like Da Vinci, who studied human anatomy and was eager to discover whether there really is a little planet within human body that may operate in the same way as the universe. The pursuit of these people's discerning eyes has eventually widened our horizon.

Perhaps, the meaning of searching is not always the result. Crossing the mountains and the rivers, one might accomplish self-cultivation little by little during the journey. May everyone of us achieve nobility and dignity of human by looking for the beauty and the truth of this world.

日 月 星 辰

THE SUN THE MOON AND THE STARS

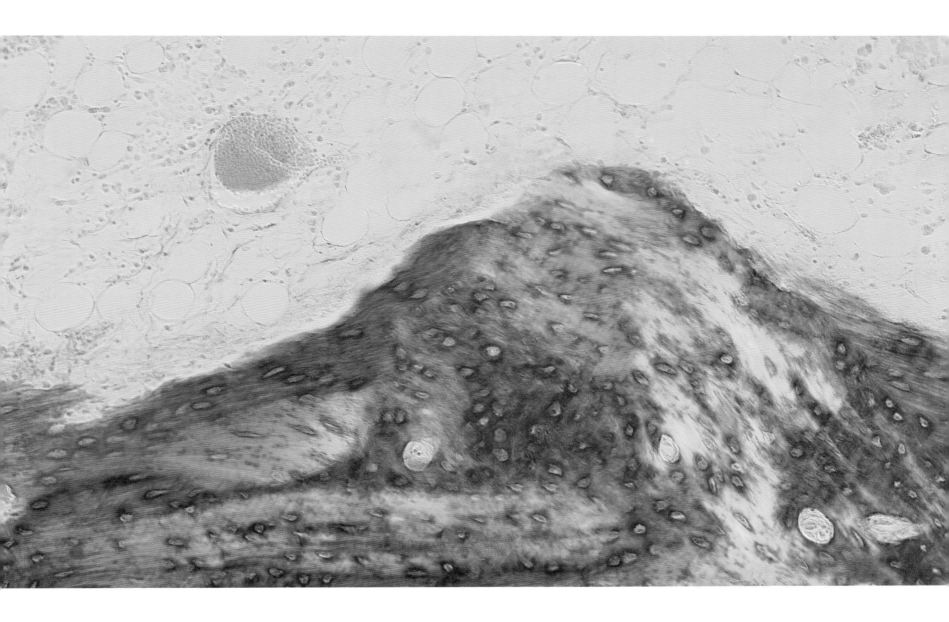

江山多娇

脱钙骨组织切片，×100，明视野 + 偏振光，2019

Beautiful Mountain

Trabecular bone, Tissue section, ×100, Light field + polarized light, 2019

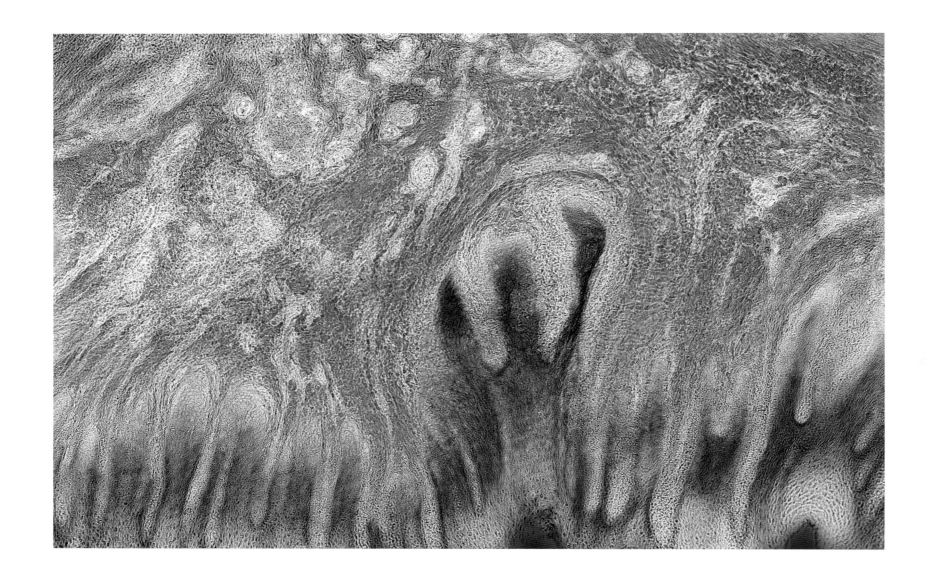

风和日丽

牙龈黏膜组织切片，×100，明视野 + 偏振光，2019

Lovely Day

Gingival mucosa, Tissue section, ×100, Light field + polarized light, 2019

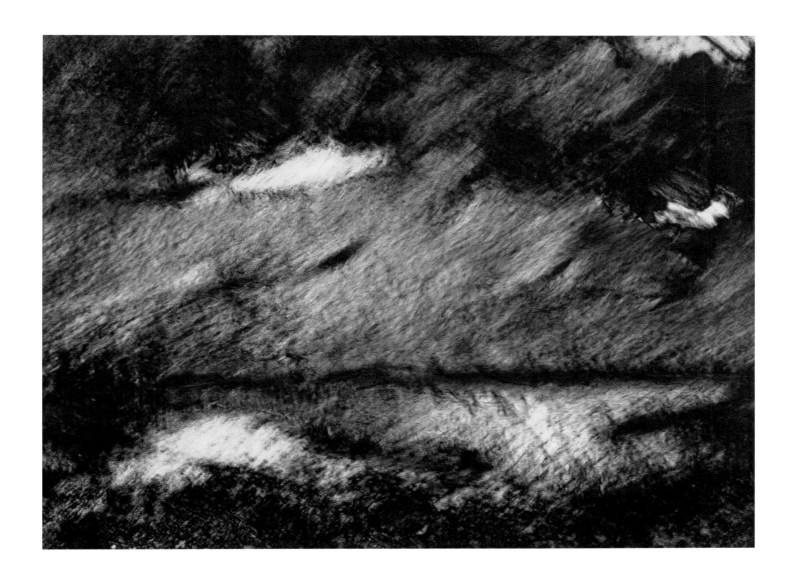

湖边午后
脱钙牙槽骨和牙周膜组织切片，×40，偏振光，2013

Sunset by the Lake
Periodontium, Combined section of jaw bone, ×40, Polarized light, 2013

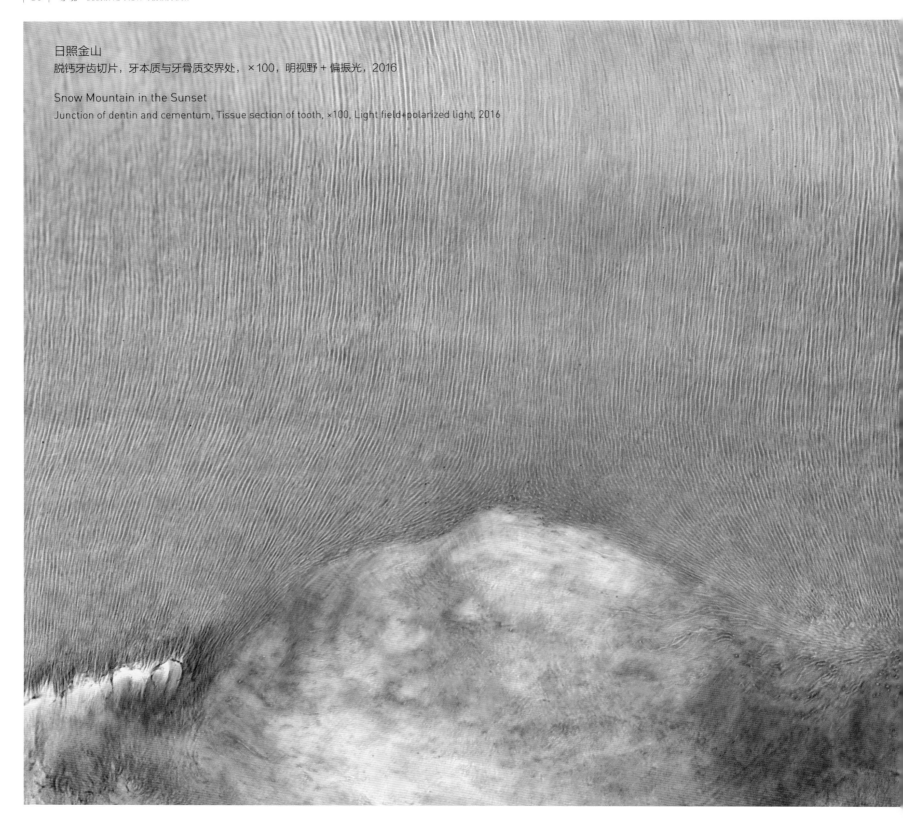

日照金山
脱钙牙齿切片，牙本质与牙骨质交界处，×100，明视野＋偏振光，2016

Snow Mountain in the Sunset
Junction of dentin and cementum, Tissue section of tooth, ×100, Light field+polarized light, 2016

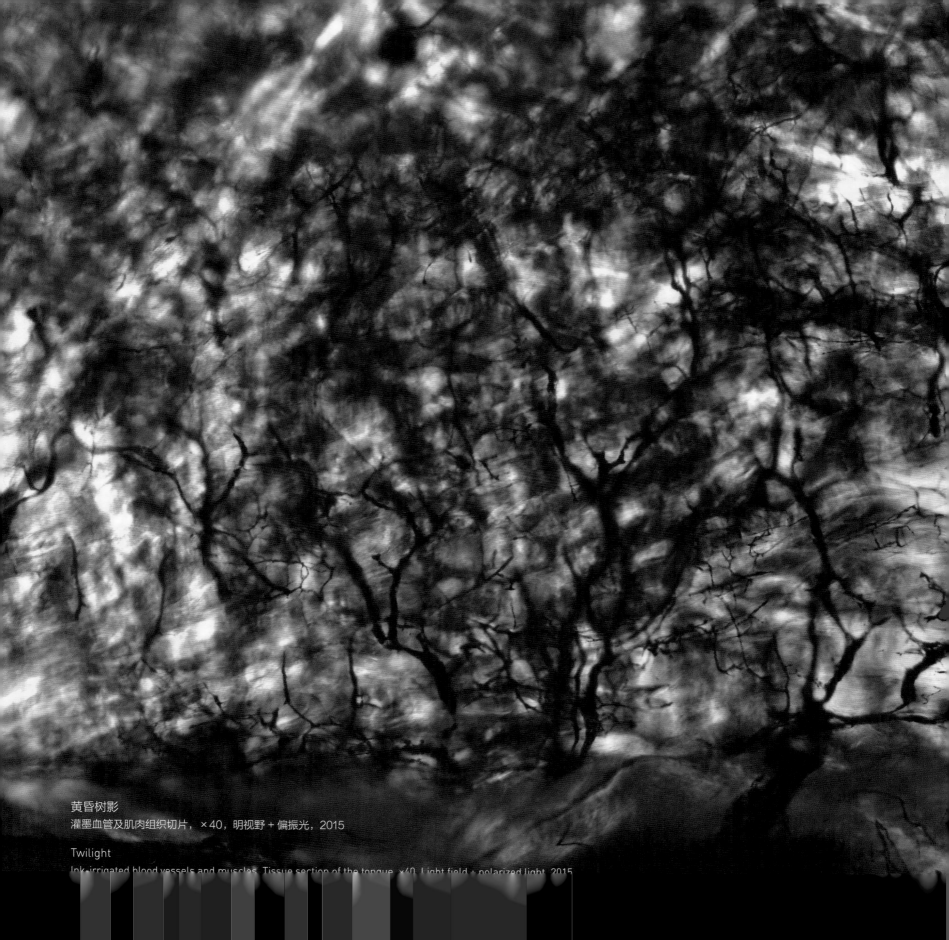

黄昏树影

灌墨血管及肌肉组织切片，×40，明视野＋偏振光，2015

Twilight

Ink-irrigated blood vessels and muscles. Tissue section of the tongue, ×40, Light field + polarized light, 2015

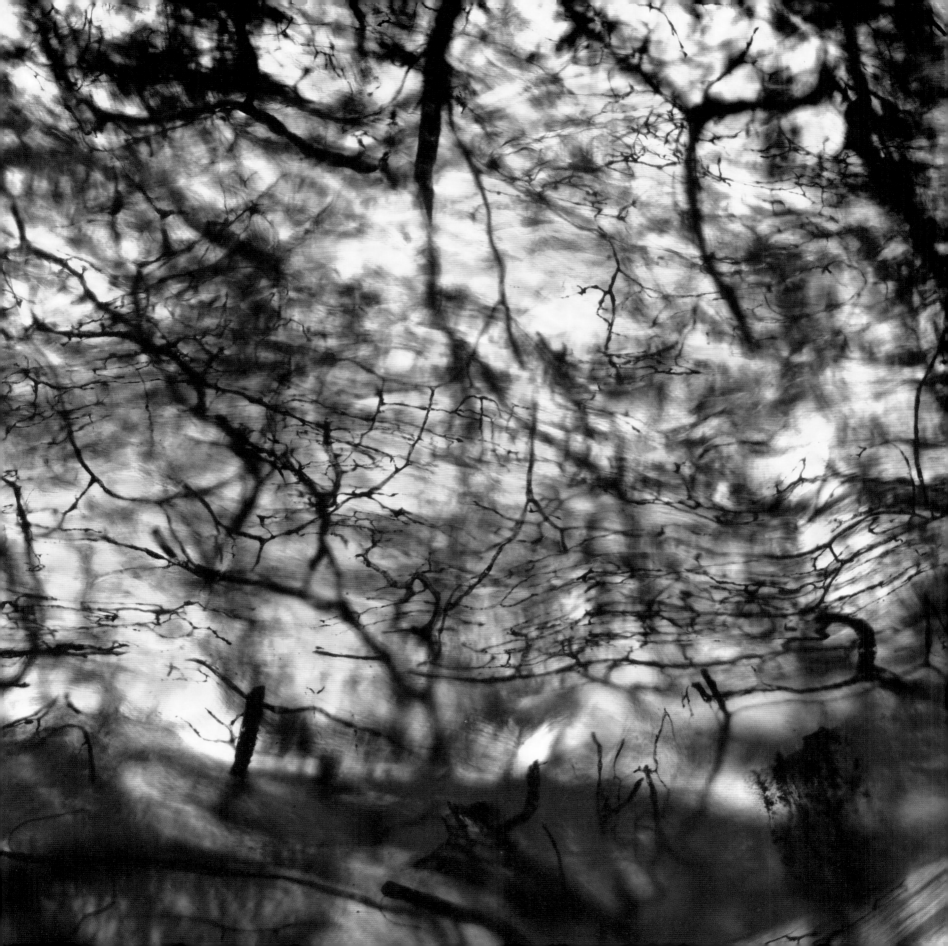

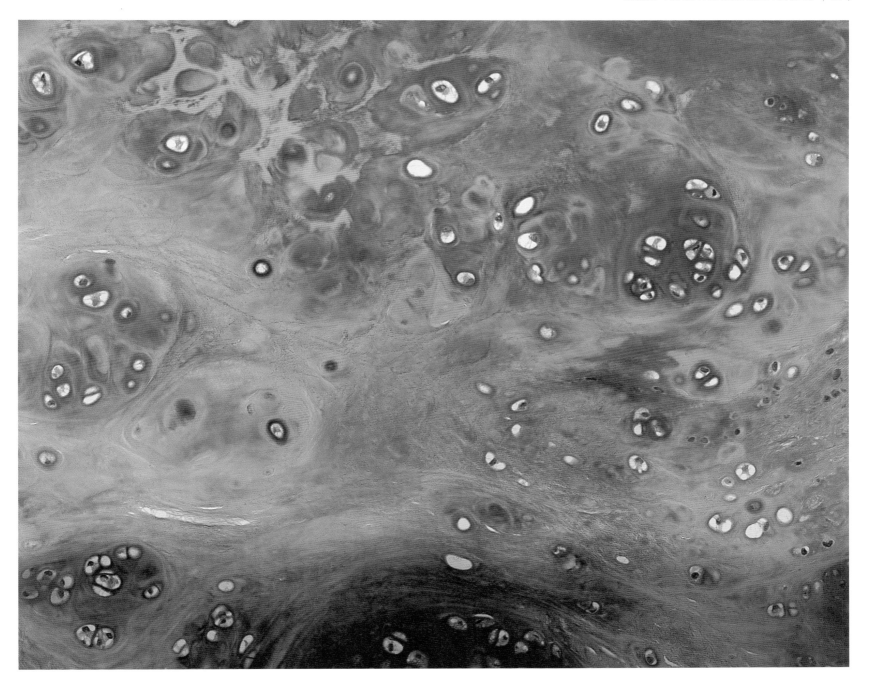

月色星光
软骨组织切片，×100，明视野 + 偏振光，2019

Stars in the Moon Light
Cartilage, Tissue section, ×100, Light field + polarized light, 2019

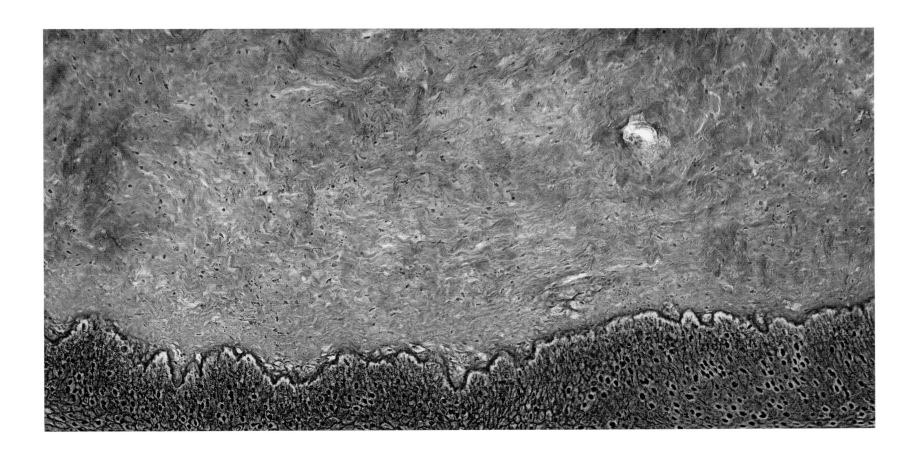

入夜
口腔黏膜上皮组织切片，×40，明视野 + 偏振光，2017

Into the Night
Oral mucosa, Tissue section, ×40, Light field + polarized light, 2017

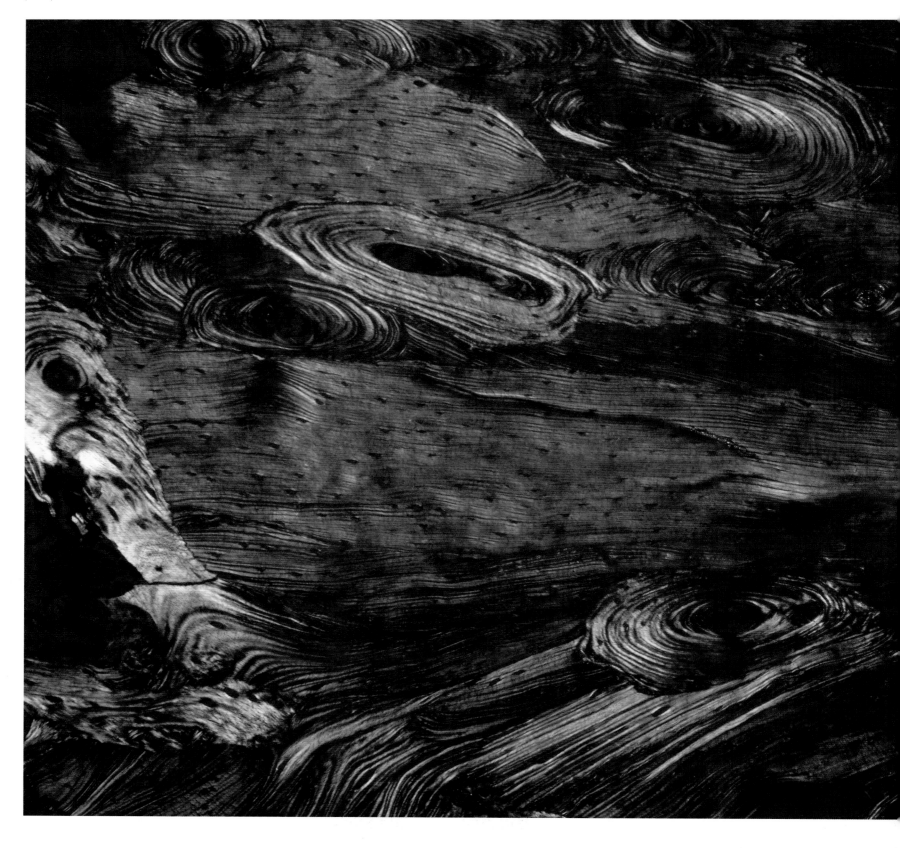

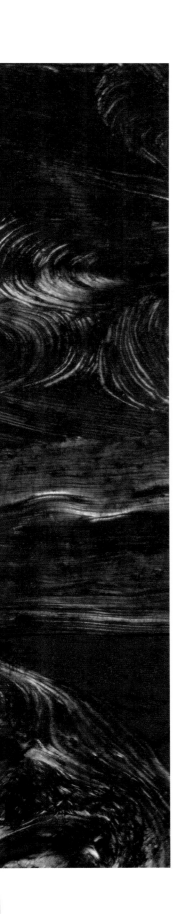

夜色
脱钙骨组织切片，×100，偏振光，2014

Night Sky
Cortical bone, Tissue section, ×100, Polarized light, 2014

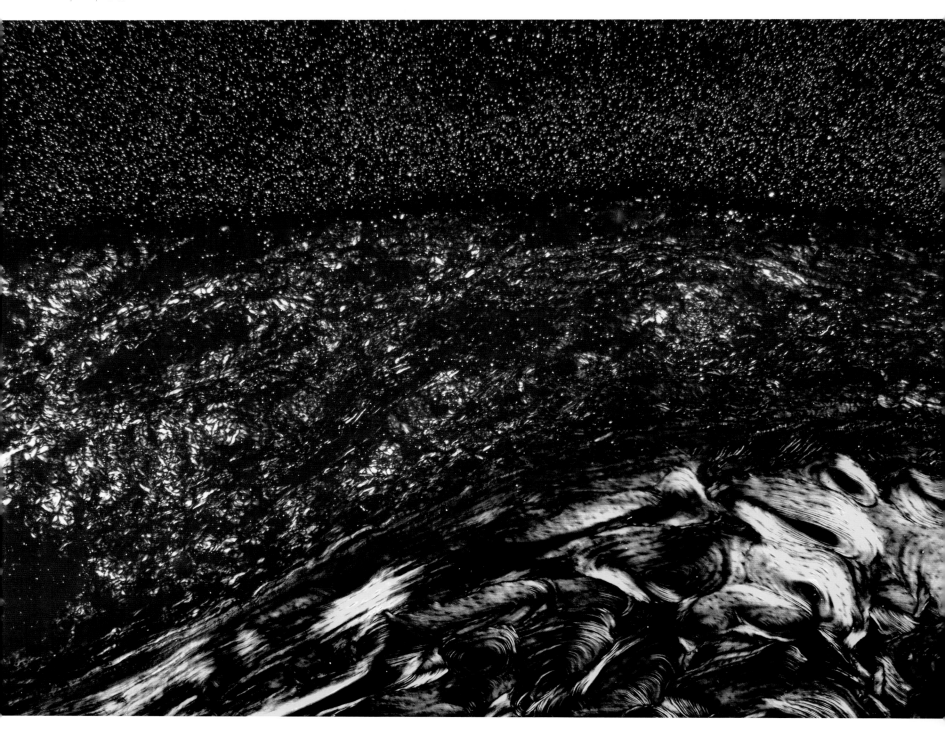

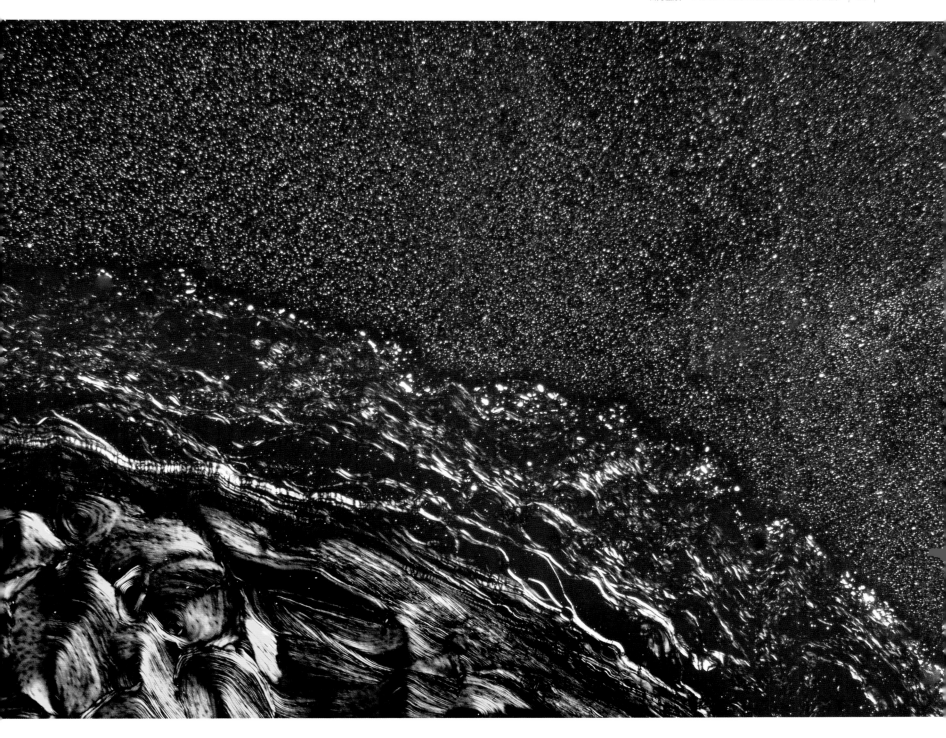

星空
脱钙骨组织切片和封片胶，×100，偏振光，2017

Starry Sky
Cortical bone and sealing glue, Tissue section, ×100, Polarized light, 2017

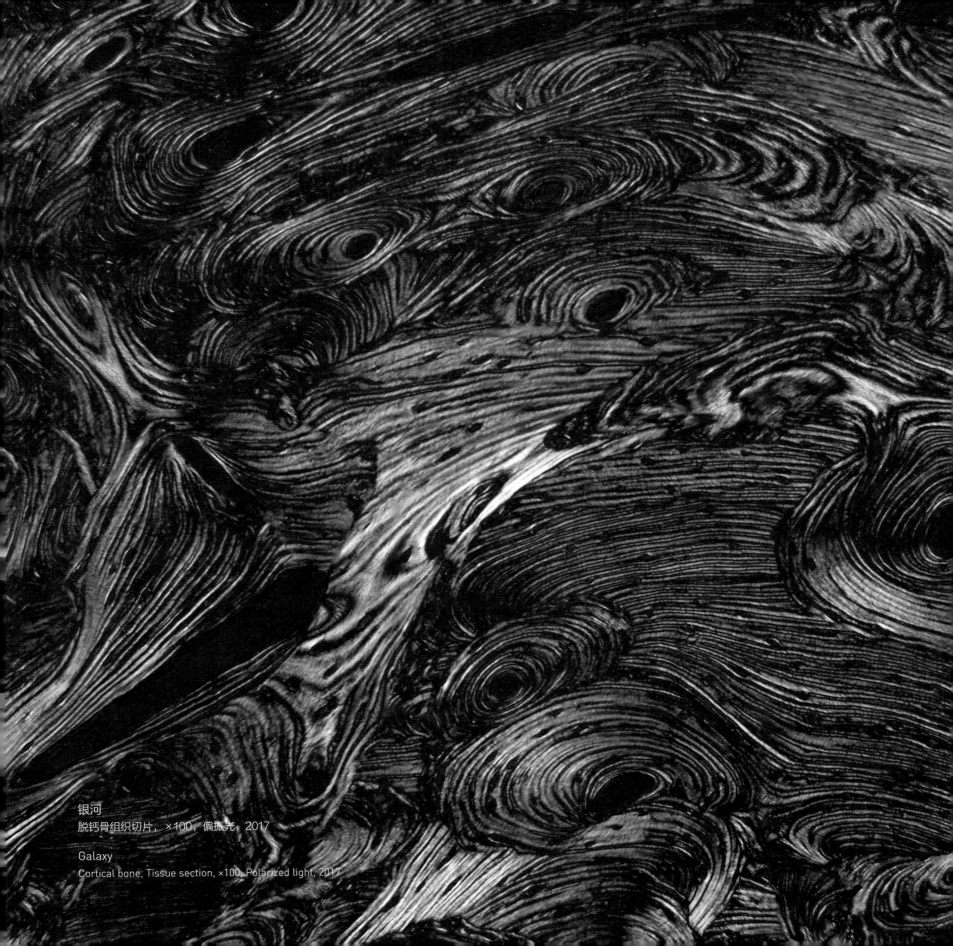

银河
脱钙骨组织切片，×100，偏振光，2017

Galaxy
Cortical bone, Tissue section, ×100, Polarized light, 2017

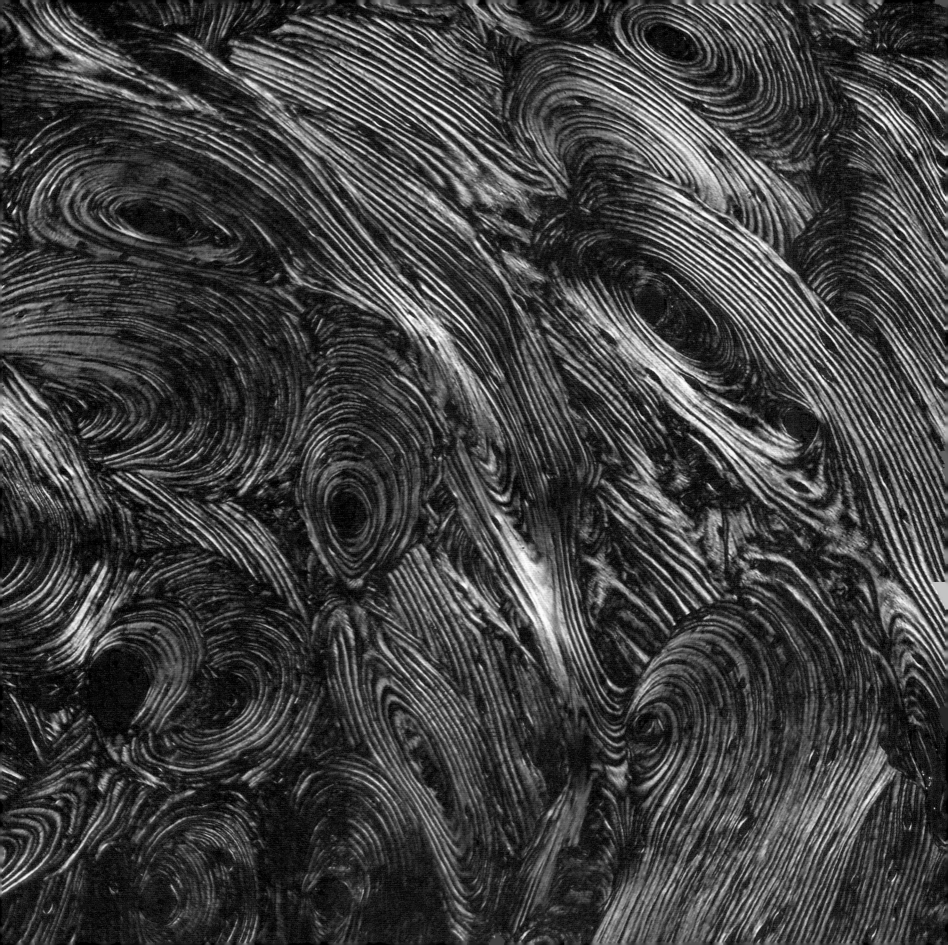

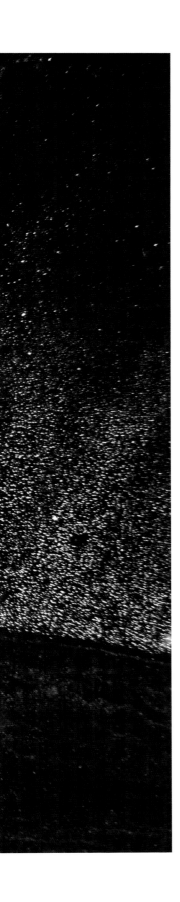

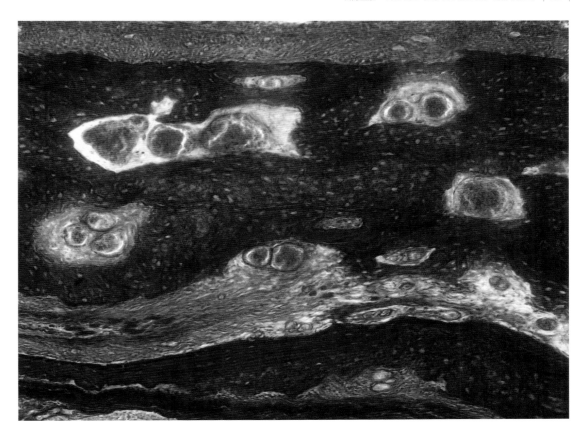

白天不懂夜的黑
脱钙骨组织切片，×200，明视野，2011

The Day Never Knows the Night's Darkness
Trabecular bone, Tissue section, ×200, Light field, 2011

火星
牙龈组织切片与封片胶交界处，×12.5，偏振光，2013

Mars
Junction between gingiva and sealing glue, Tissue section, ×12.5, Polarized light, 2013

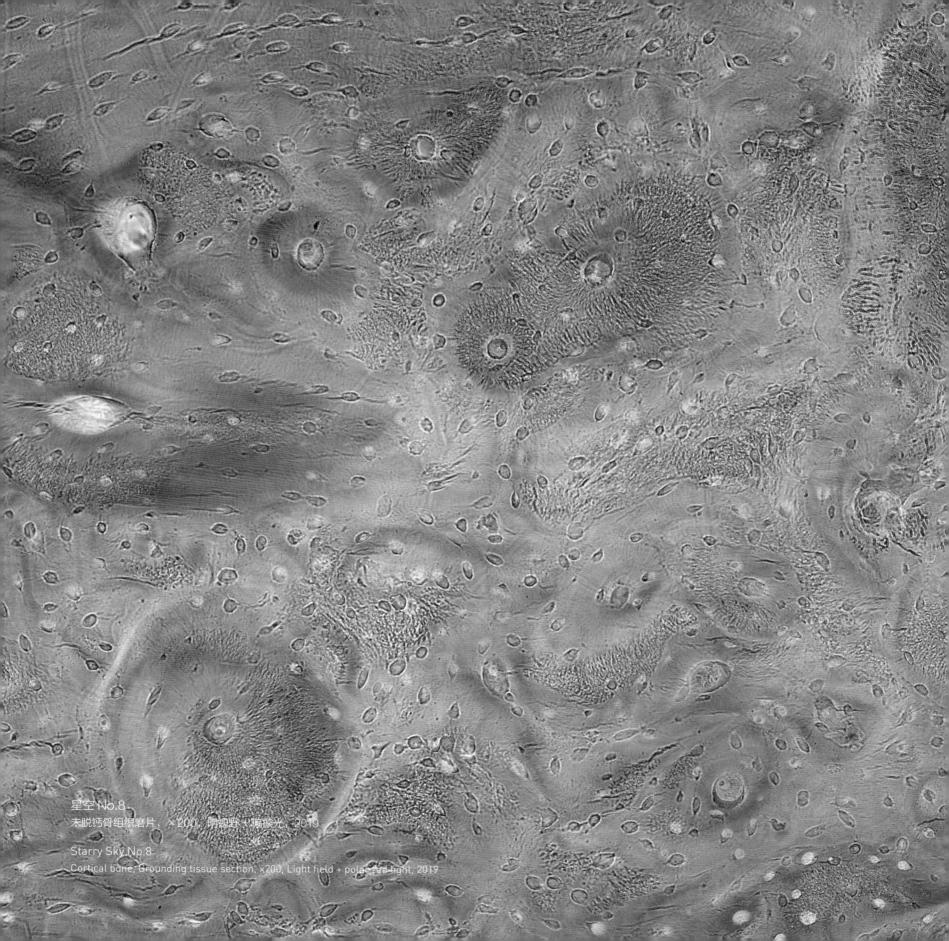

星空 No.8
未脱钙骨组织磨片，×200，明视野＋偏振光，2019

Starry Sky No.8
Cortical bone, Grounding tissue section, ×200, Light field + polarized light, 2019

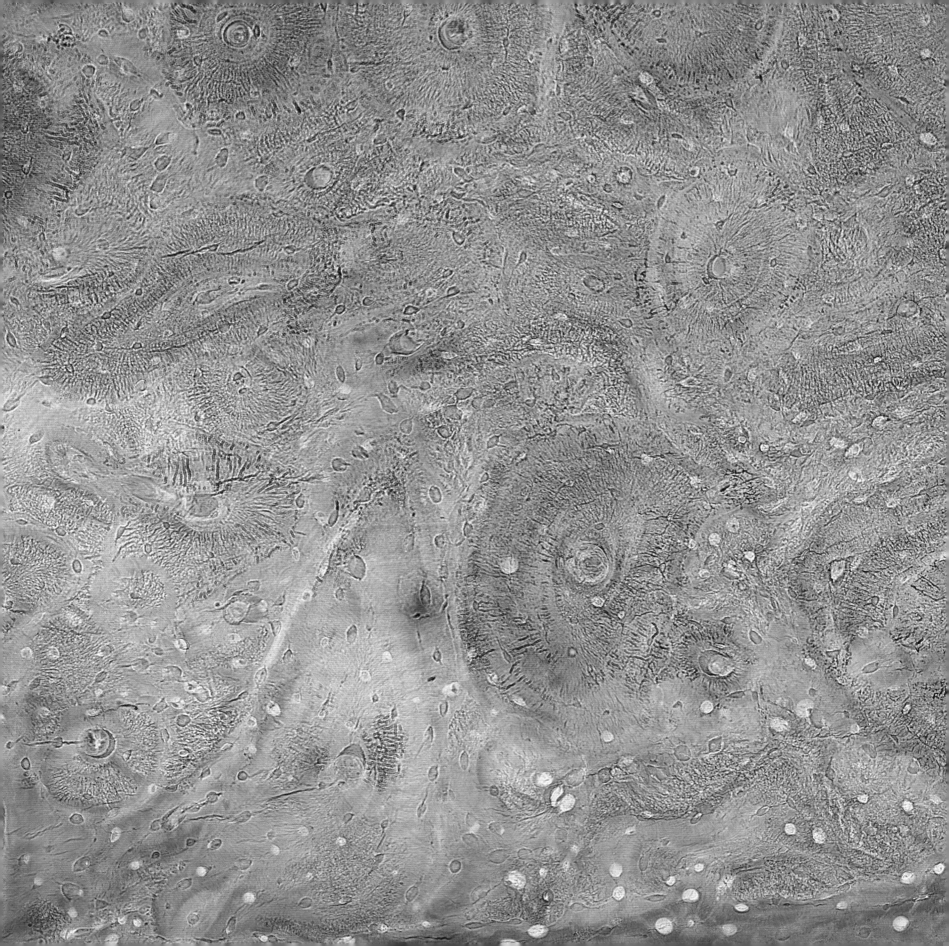

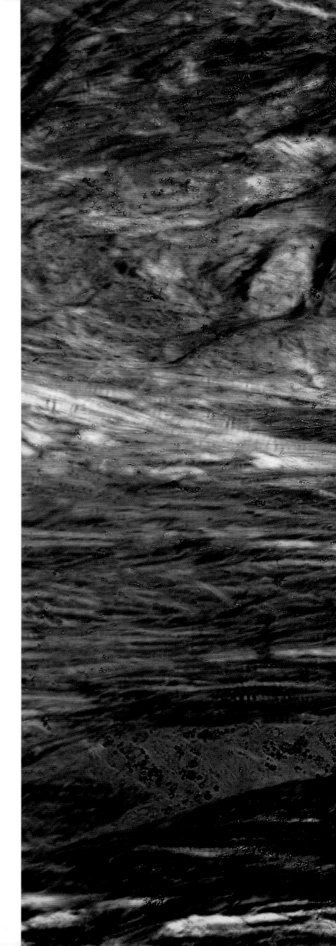

月夜
未脱钙骨磨片周围软组织，×40，偏振光，2019

Moon Night
Bone and surrounding soft tissues, Grounding tissue section, ×40, Polarized light, 2019

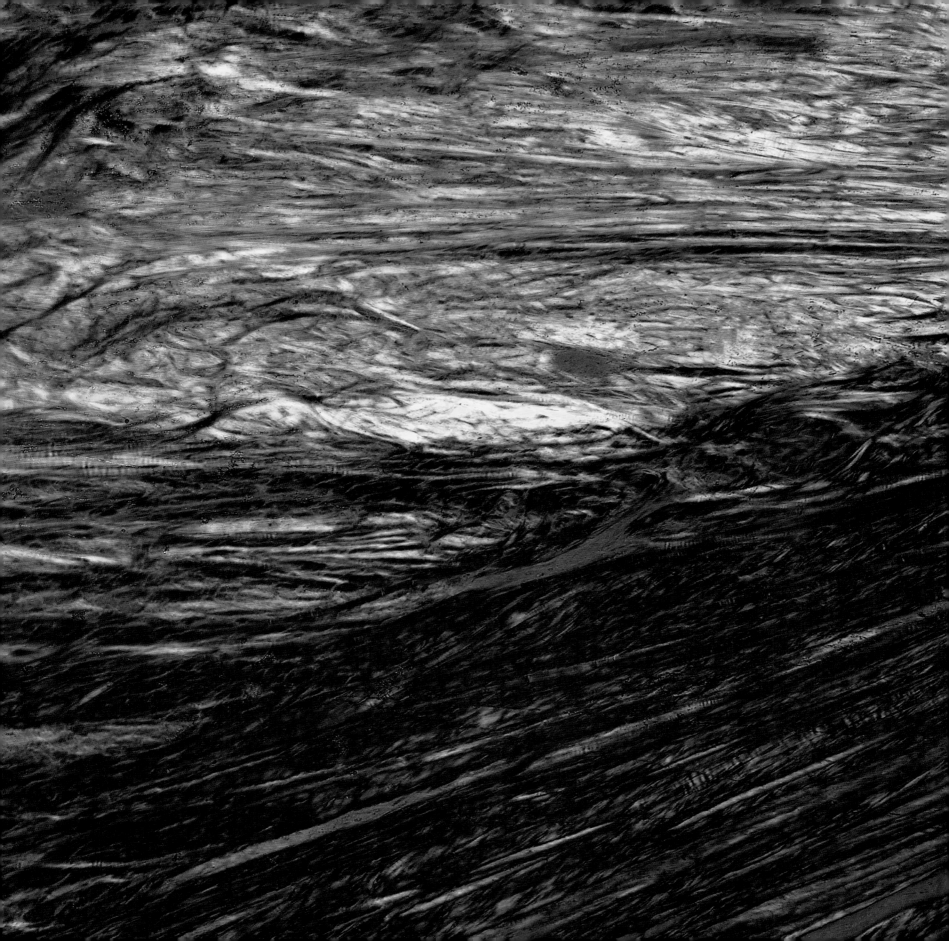

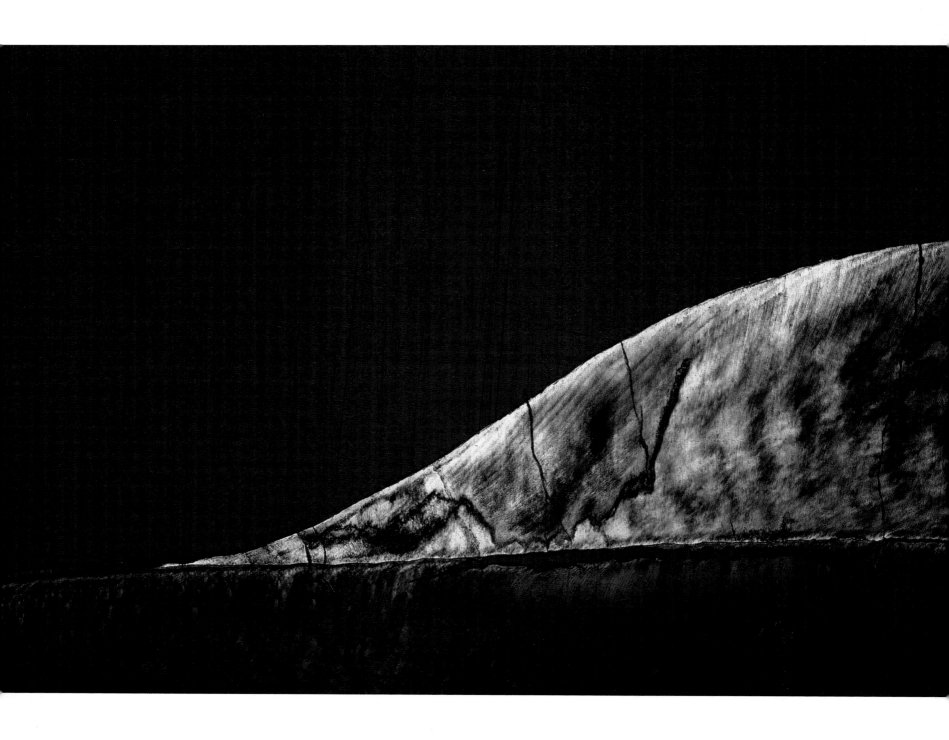

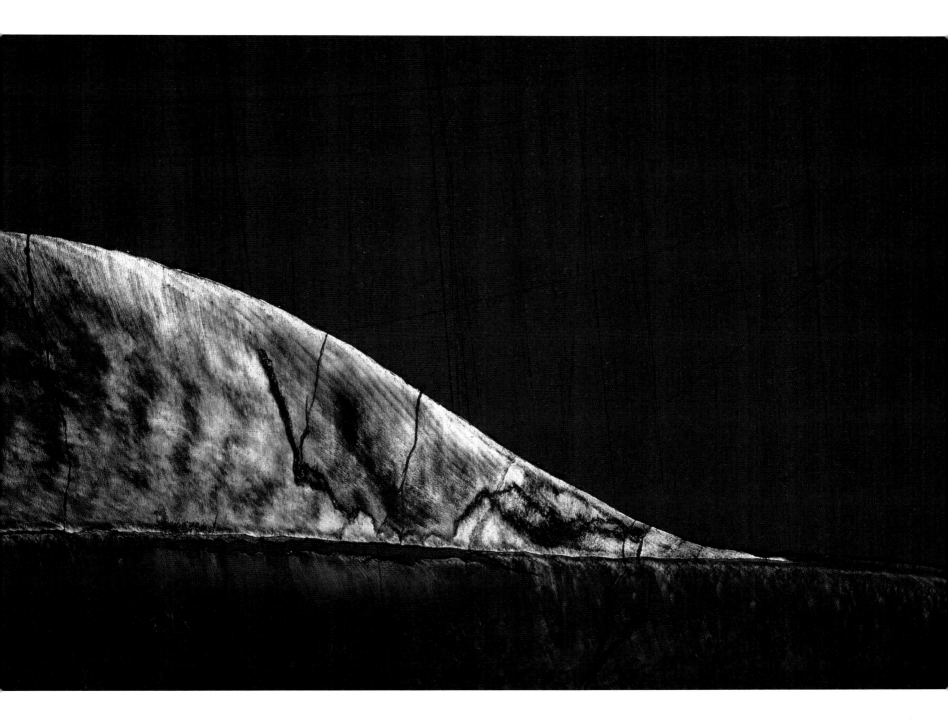

半个月亮升上来

未脱钙牙釉质磨片的局部镜像，×100，偏振光，2019

Rising Moon

Mirror image of part of enamel, Grounding tissue section, ×100, Polarized light, 2019

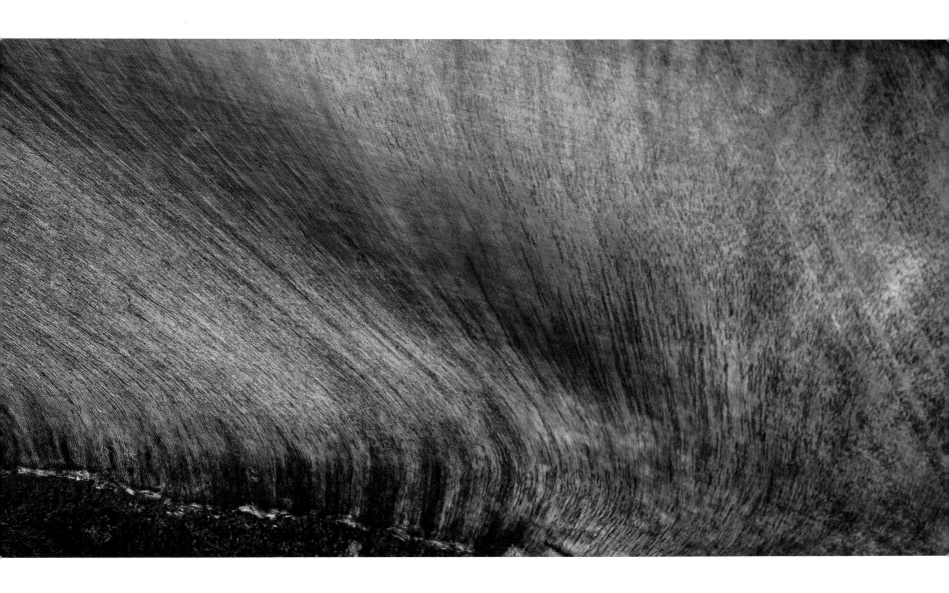

极光

未脱钙牙齿磨片牙本质组织，×200，偏振光，2019

Aurora

Dentin tissue, Grounding section, ×200, Polarized light, 2019

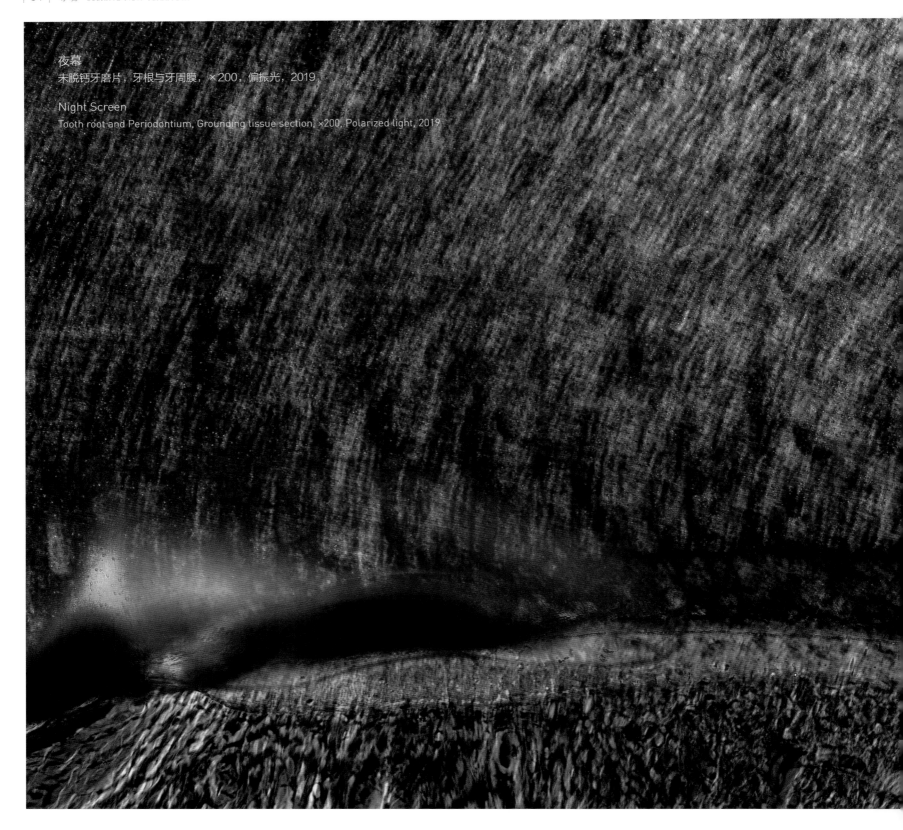

夜幕
未脱钙牙磨片，牙根与牙周膜，×200，偏振光，2019

Night Screen
Tooth root and Periodontium, Grounding tissue section, ×200, Polarized light, 2019

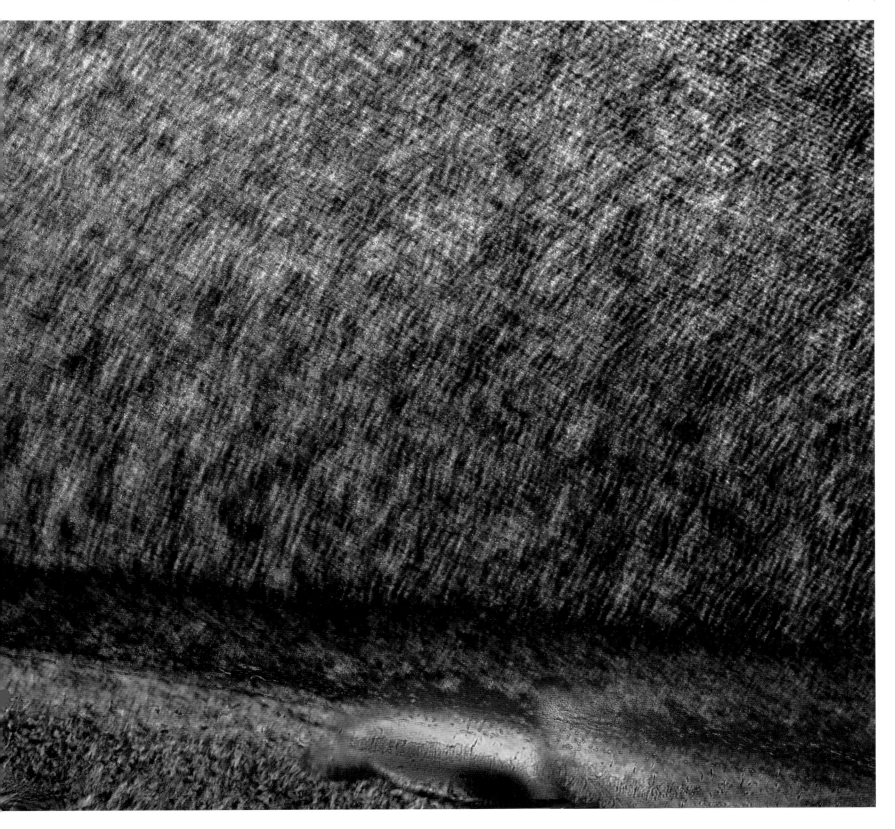

四季大地

Landscapes of the Four Seasons

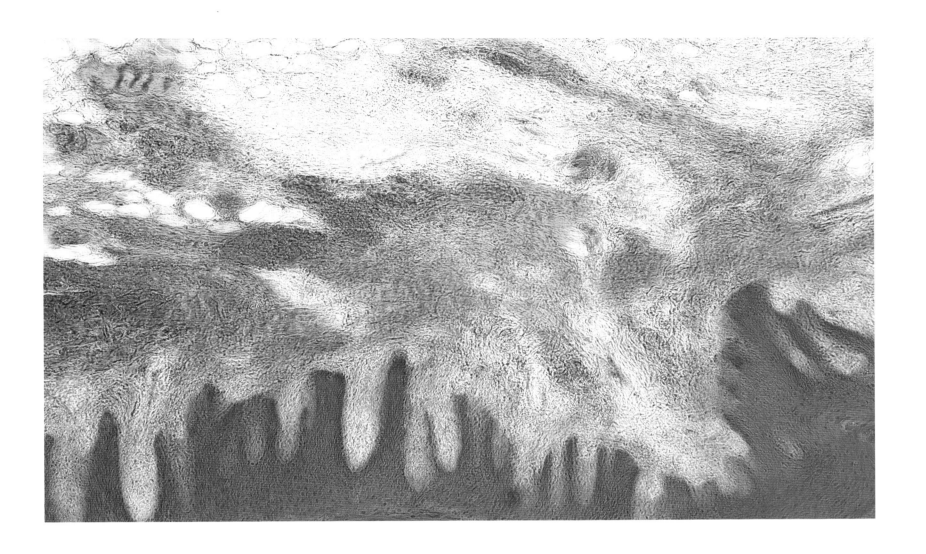

土林霞光

牙龈黏膜组织切片，×40，明视野，2016

Pink Clouds Over Earth Forest

Gingival mucosa, Tissue section, ×40, Light field, 2016

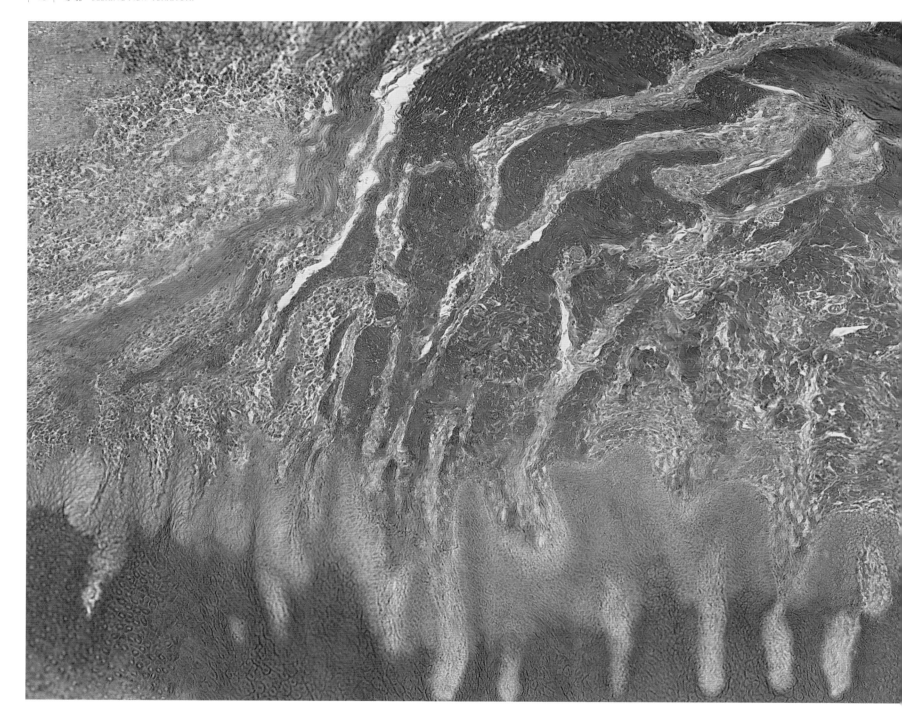

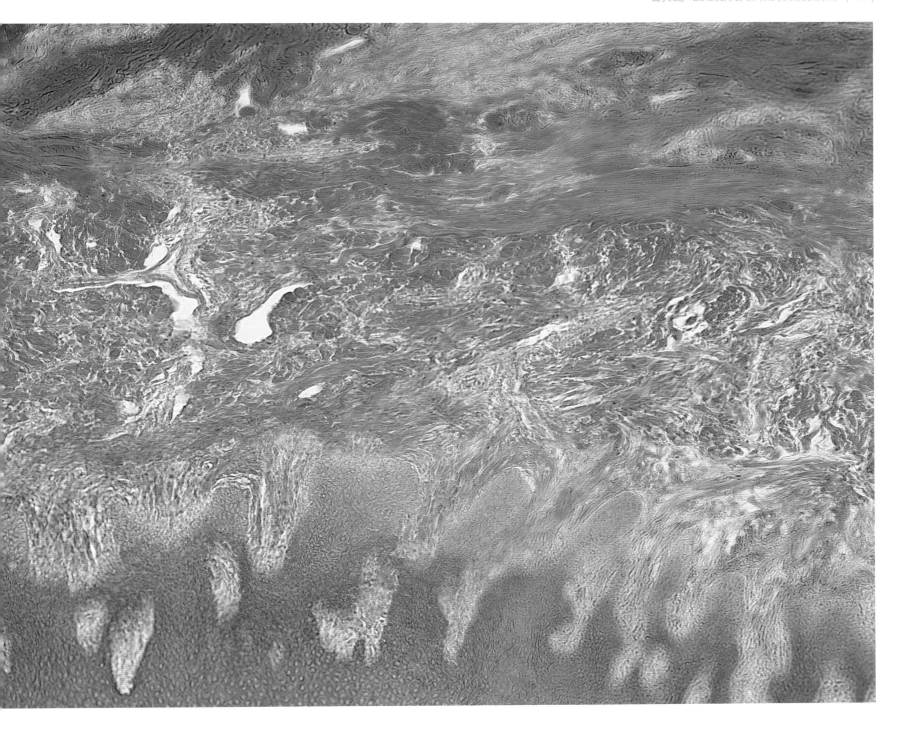

飘

牙龈组织切片，×100，明视野，2016

Gone with the Wind

Gingival mucosa, Tissue section, ×100, Light field, 2016

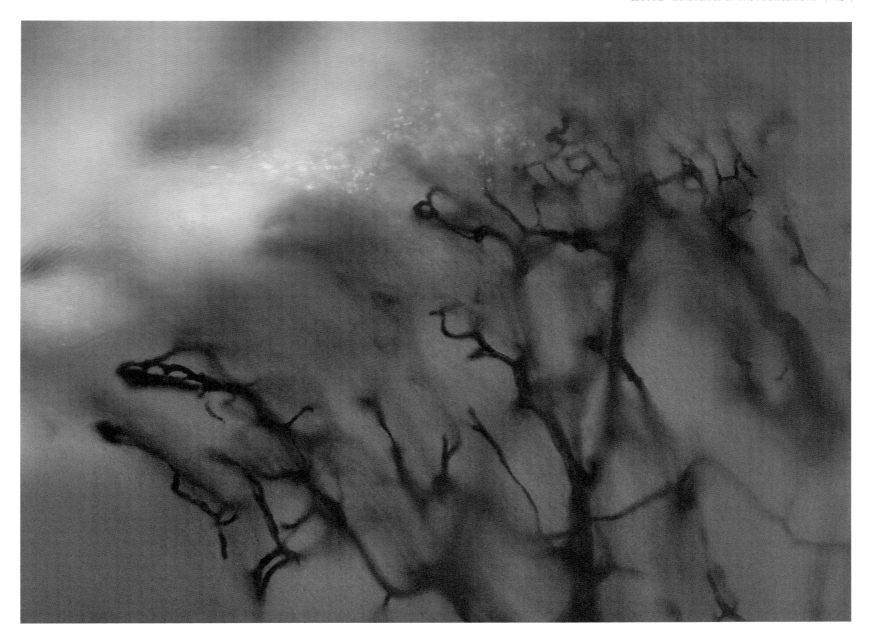

春雨
灌墨血管组织切片，×100，明视野（长时间曝光），2019

The Spring Rain
Ink-irrigated blood vessels, Tissue section, ×100, Light field (long exposure), 2019

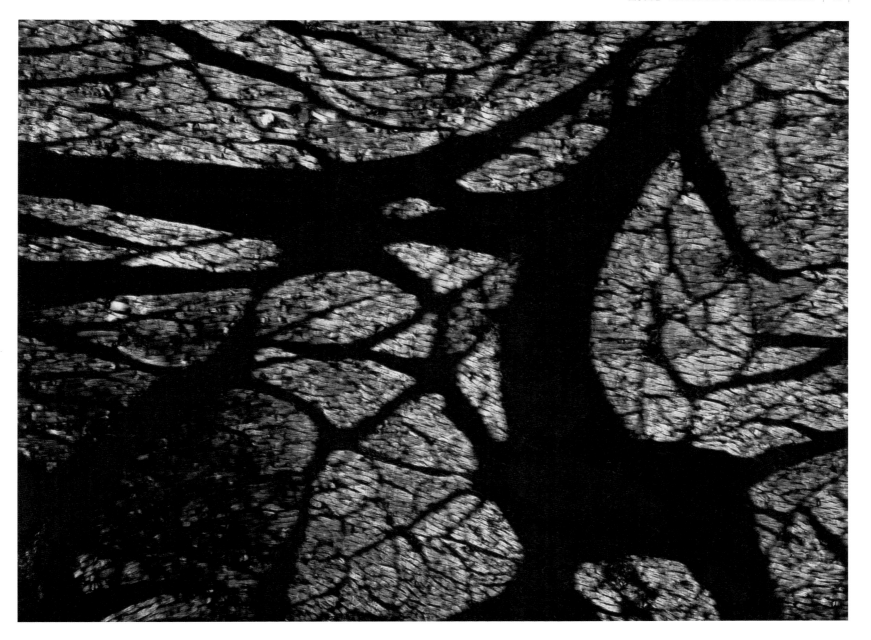

夏日

横纹肌组织切片，×40，偏振光，2019

Summer

Striated muscle, Tissue section, ×40, Polarized light, 2019

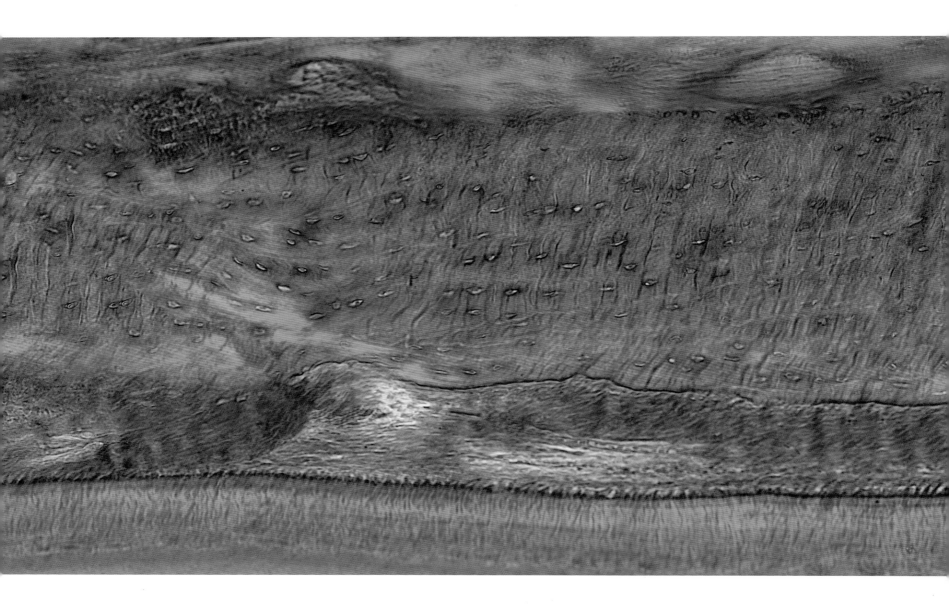

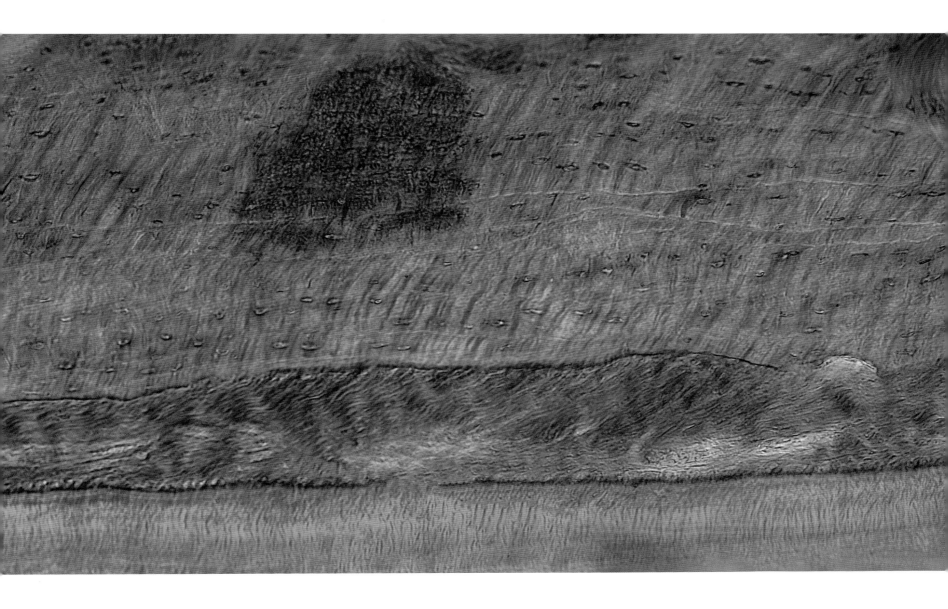

红土地
牙周组织联合切片，×100，明视野，2019

Red Land
Periodontium, Combined section of tooth and jaw, ×100, Light field, 2019

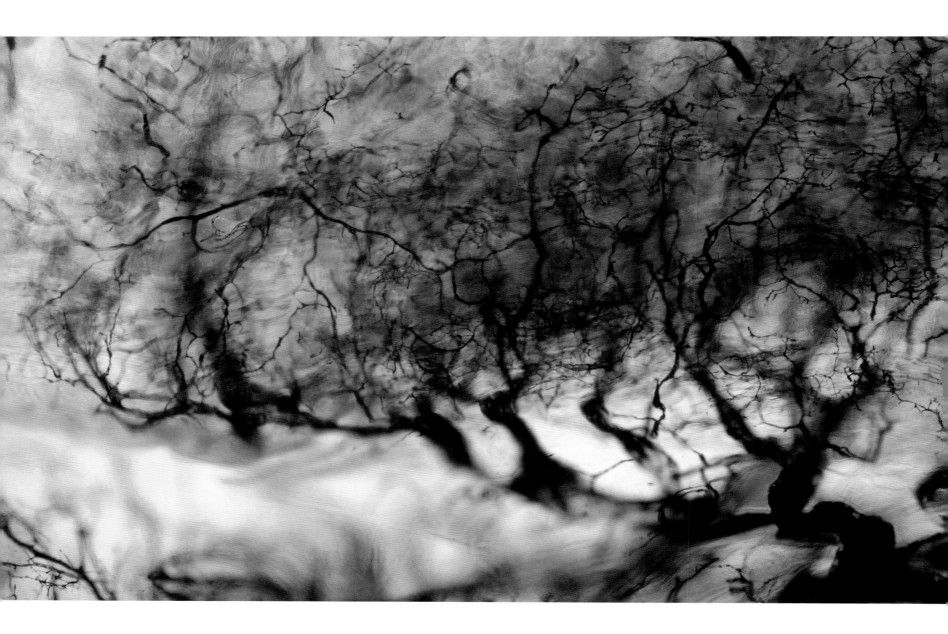

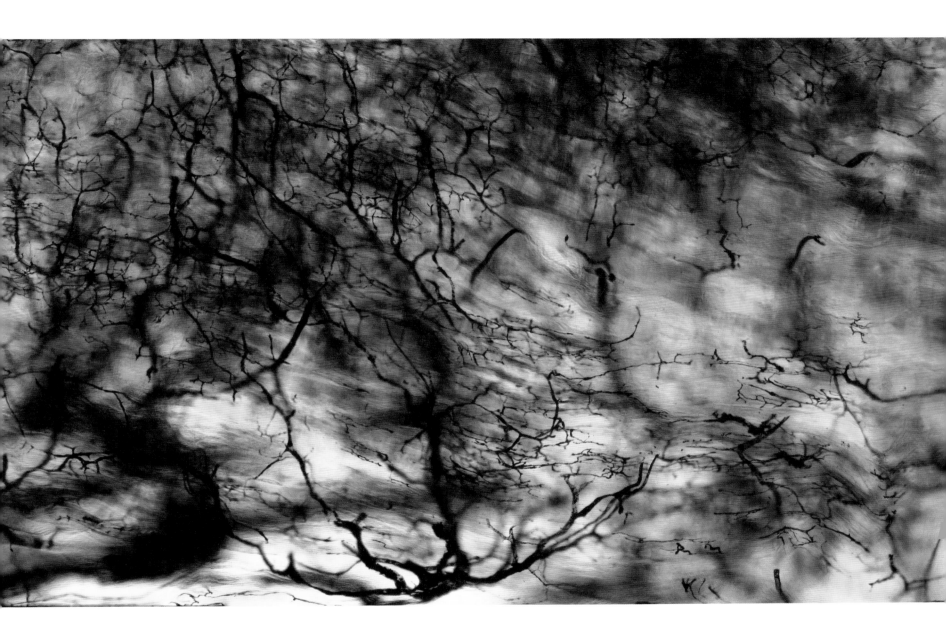

溪畔秋树

灌墨血管组织切片，×40，明视野＋偏振光，2014

Autumn Tree by the Creek

Ink-irrigated blood vessels, Tissue section, ×40, Light field + polarized light, 2014

满山红遍
上皮角质组织切片，×100，明视野，2011

Autumn Clour of Mountains
Keratinized materials of epithelium, Tissue section, ×100, Light field, 2011

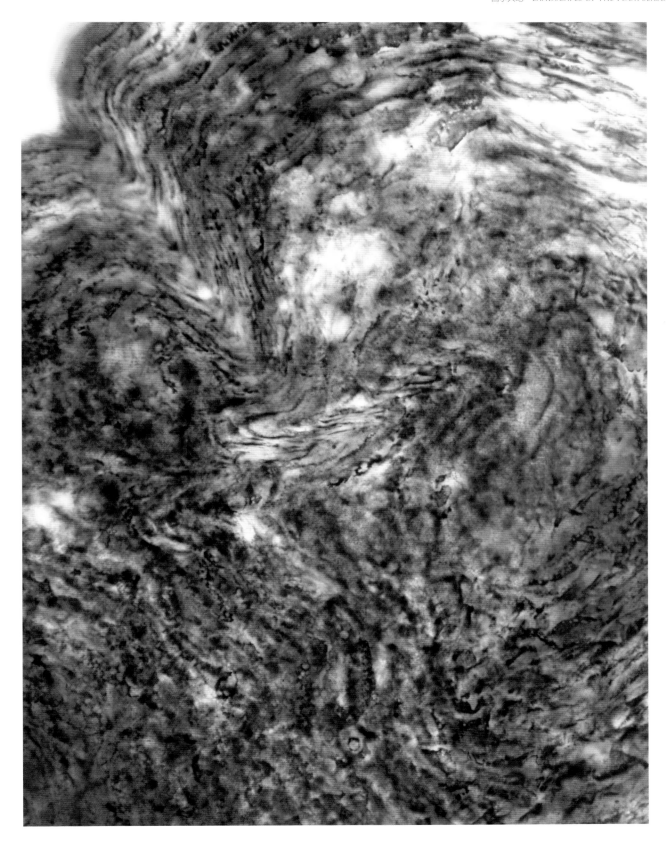

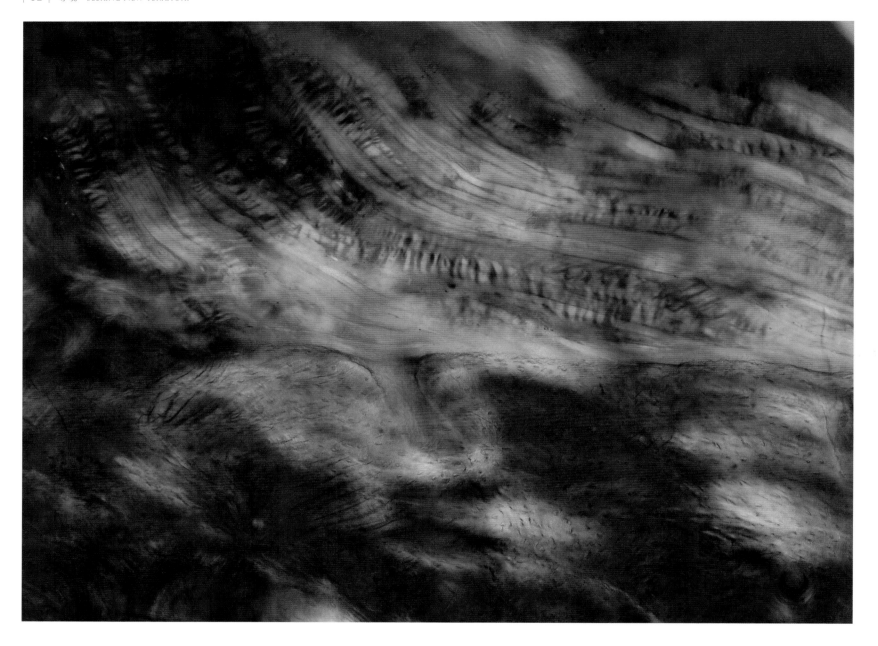

晚秋

骨组织和肌肉组织切片，×100，明视野 + 偏振光，2013

Late Autumn

Bone and muscel, Tissue section, ×100, Light field + polarized light, 2013

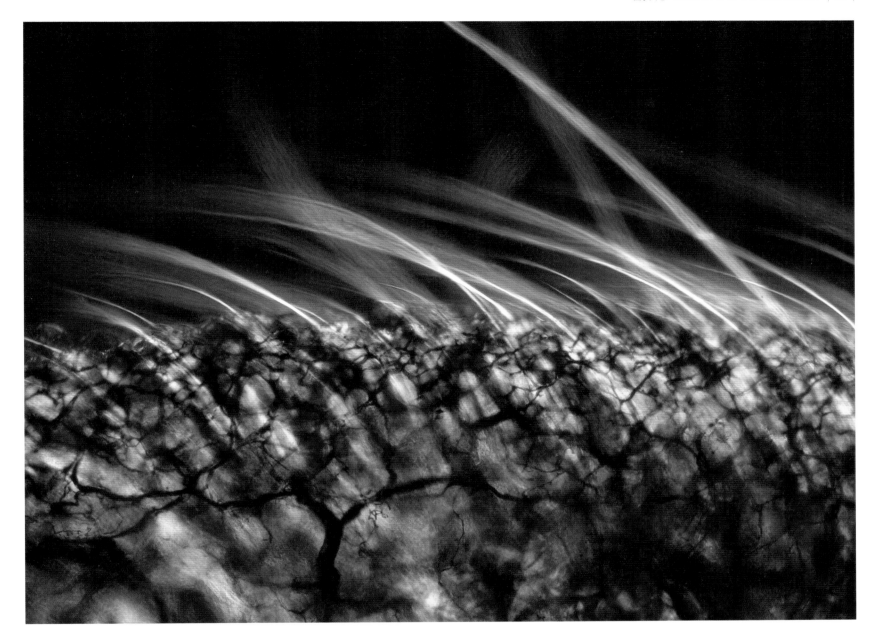

晚风
皮肤及毛发组织切片，×12.5，偏振光，2016

Evening Wind
Skin with hair, Tissue section, ×12.5, Polarized light, 2016

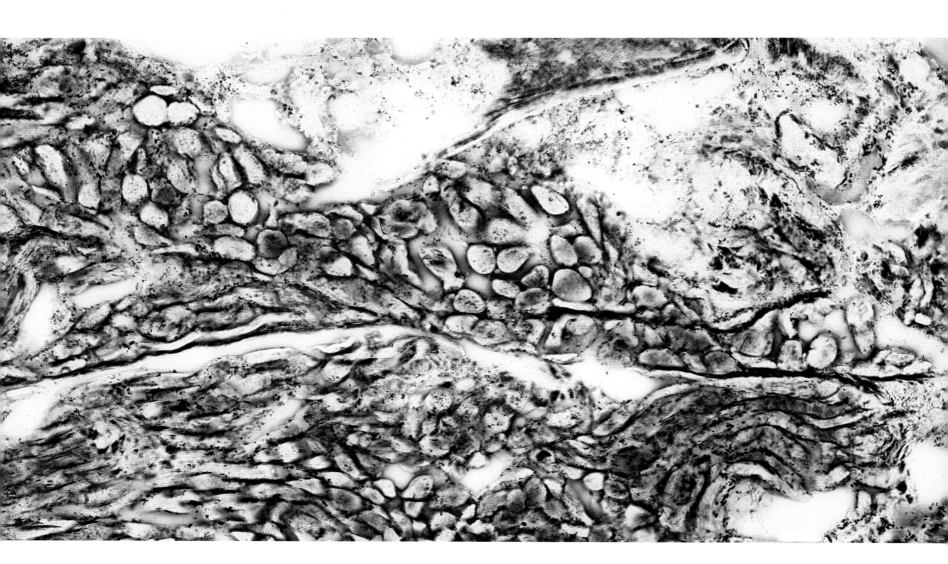

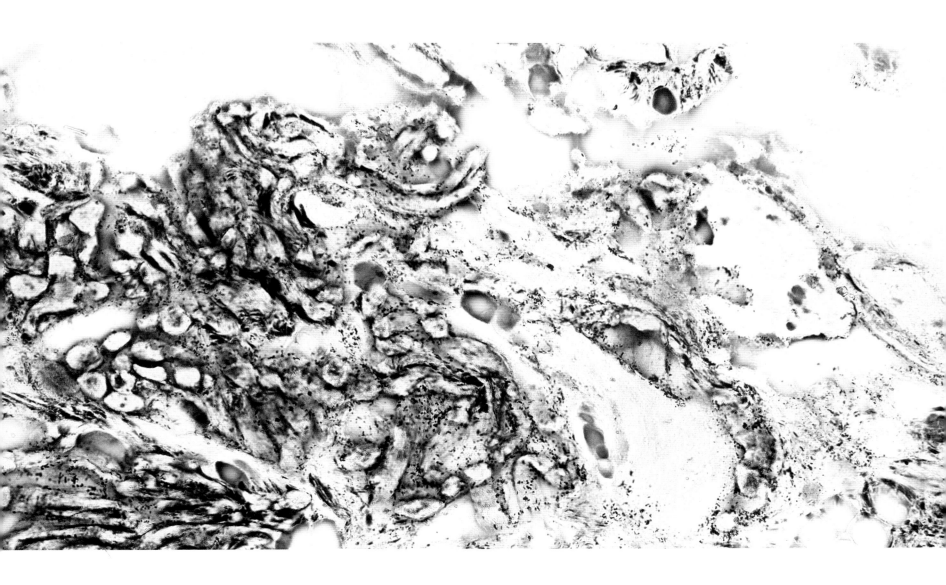

寒山长卷

银染横纹肌组织切片，×200 ，明视野，2017

Snow Mountain
Striated muscle, Tissue scetion, ×200, Light field, 2017

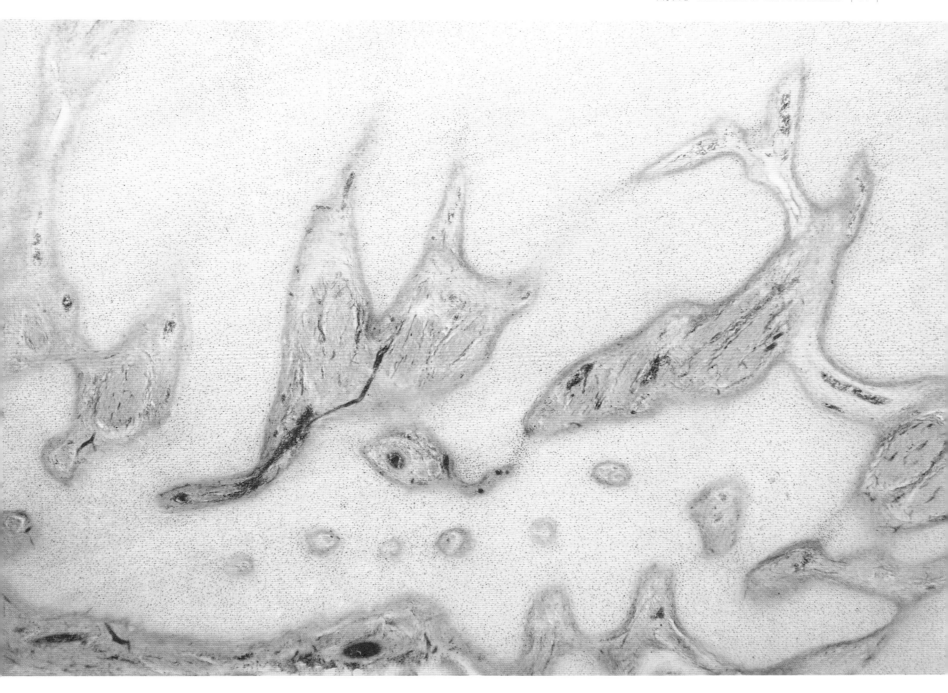

风雪
发育中的软骨组织切片，×12.5，明视野，2012

Windy Snow
Developing cartilage, Tissue section, ×12.5, Light field, 2012

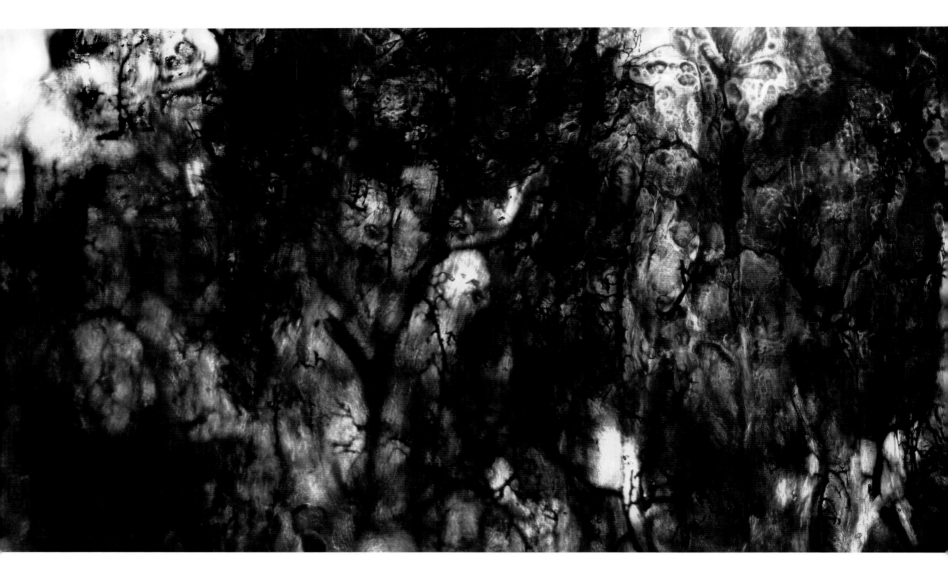

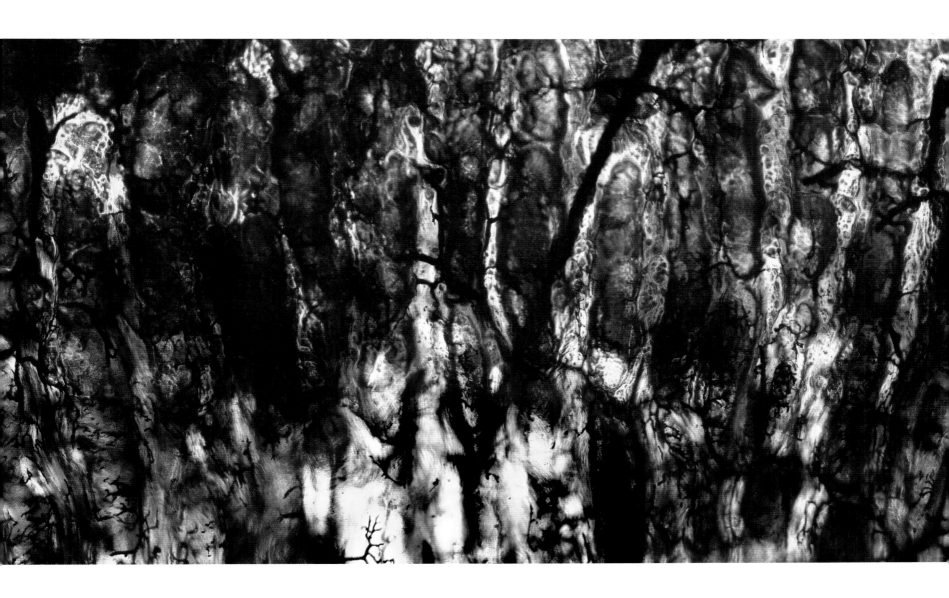

原始森林

灌墨血管及肌肉组织切片和表面的封片胶，×40，明视野 + 偏振光，2016

Primeval Forest

Ink-irrigated blood vessels and muscles with sealing glue , Tissue section, ×40, Light field + polarized light, 2016

秋林
灌墨血管及肌肉组织切片，×40，明视野，2019

Autumn Trees
Ink-irrigated blood vessels and muscles, Tissue section, ×40, Light field, 2019

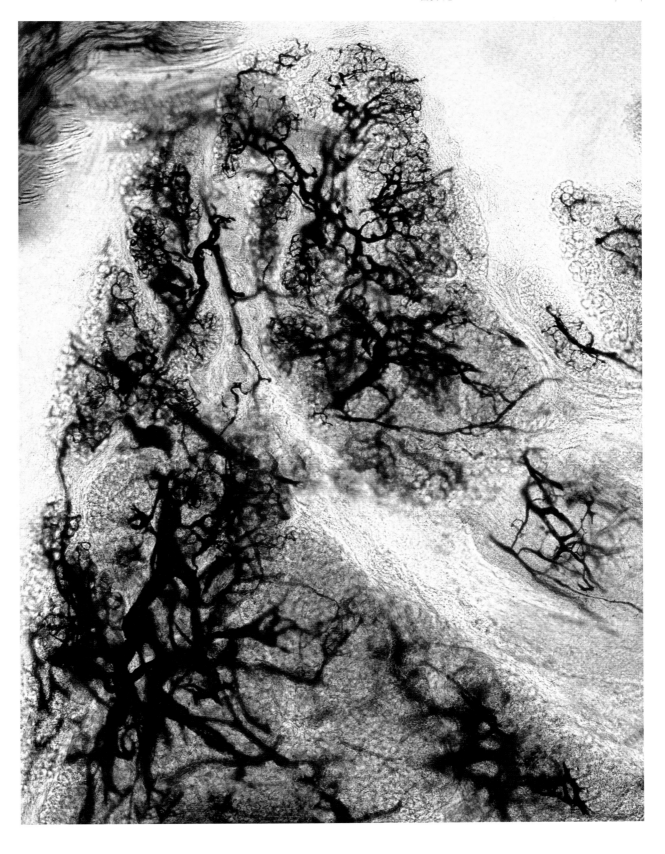

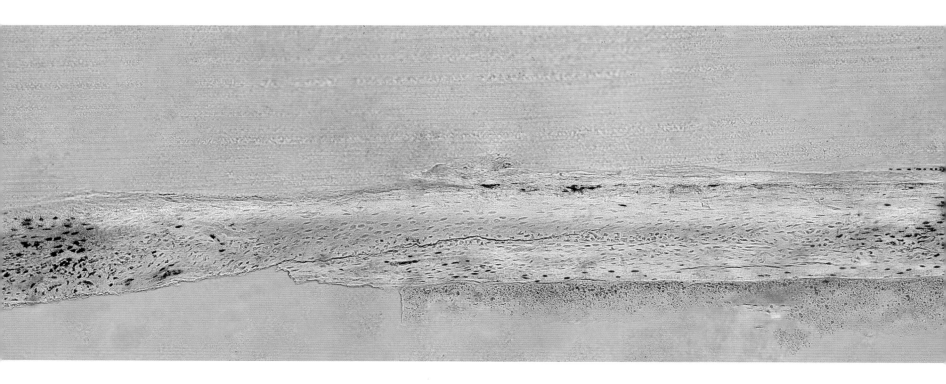

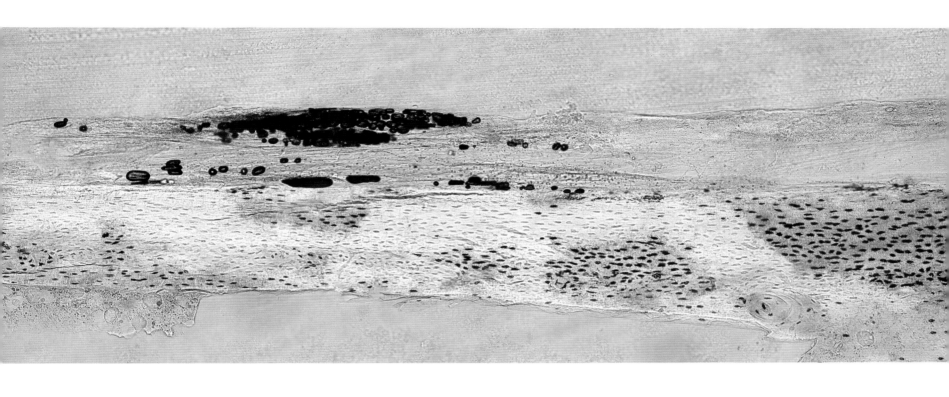

雪原
未脱钙骨组织与人工填料磨片，×100，明视野 + 偏振光，2019

Snowfield
Bone tissue with implanted materials, Grounding tissue section, ×100, Light field + polarized light, 2019

春梦
灌墨血管组织切片，×100，明视野（长时间曝光），2012

Spring Dream
Ink-irrigated blood vessels, Tissue section, ×100, Light field (long exposure), 2012

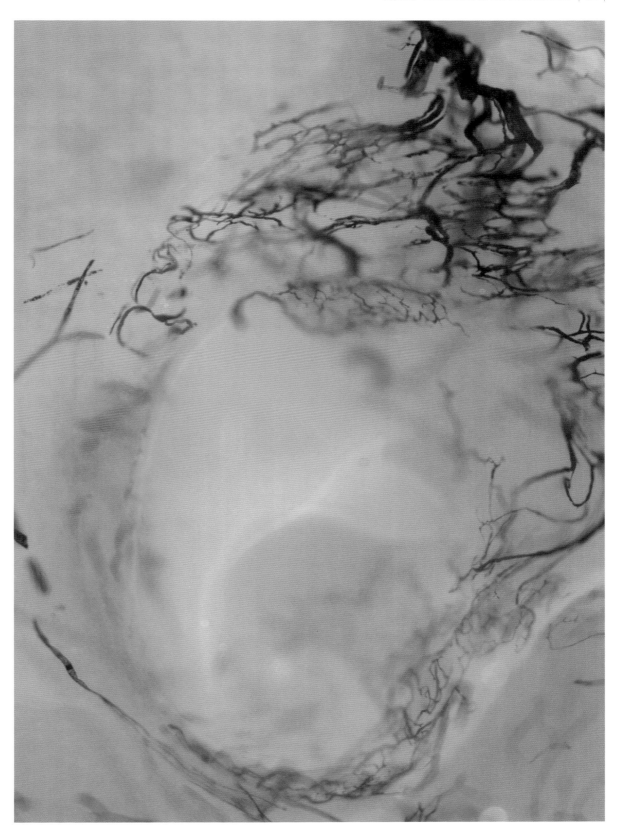

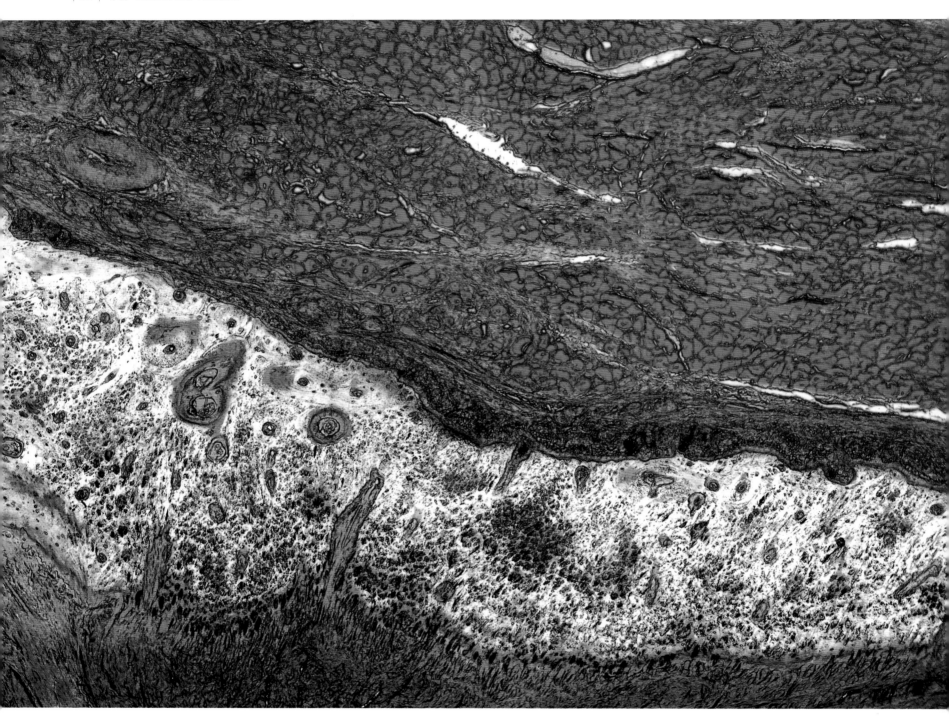

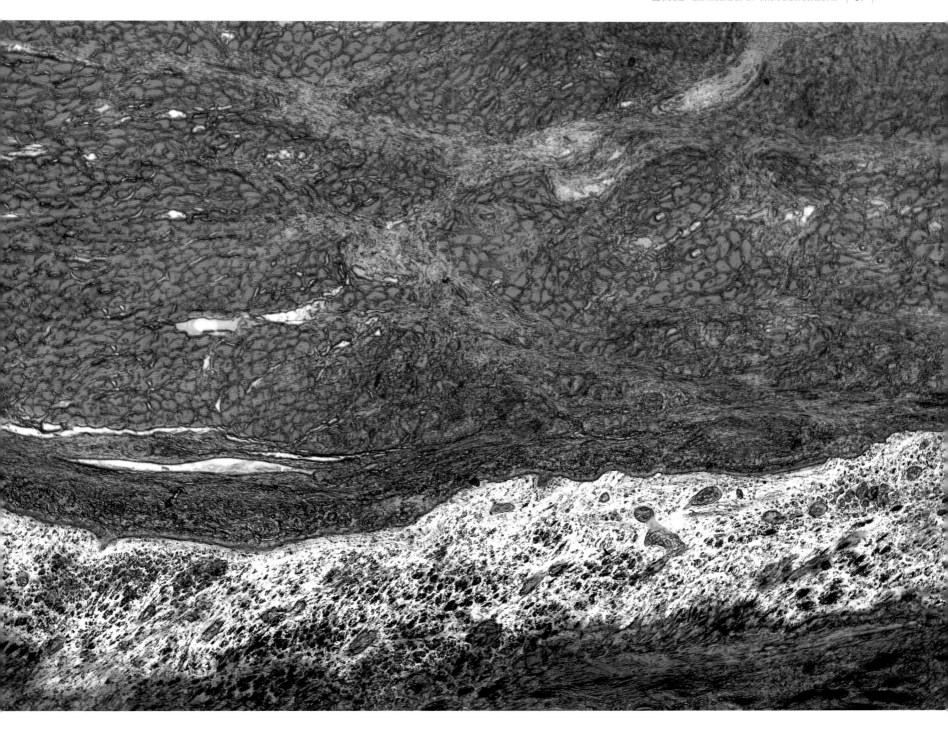

秋色漫山
未脱钙骨及肌肉组织磨片，×40，明视野 + 偏振光，2019

Autumn Painted Mountains
Bone and muscles, Grounding tissue section, ×40, Light field + polarized light, 2019

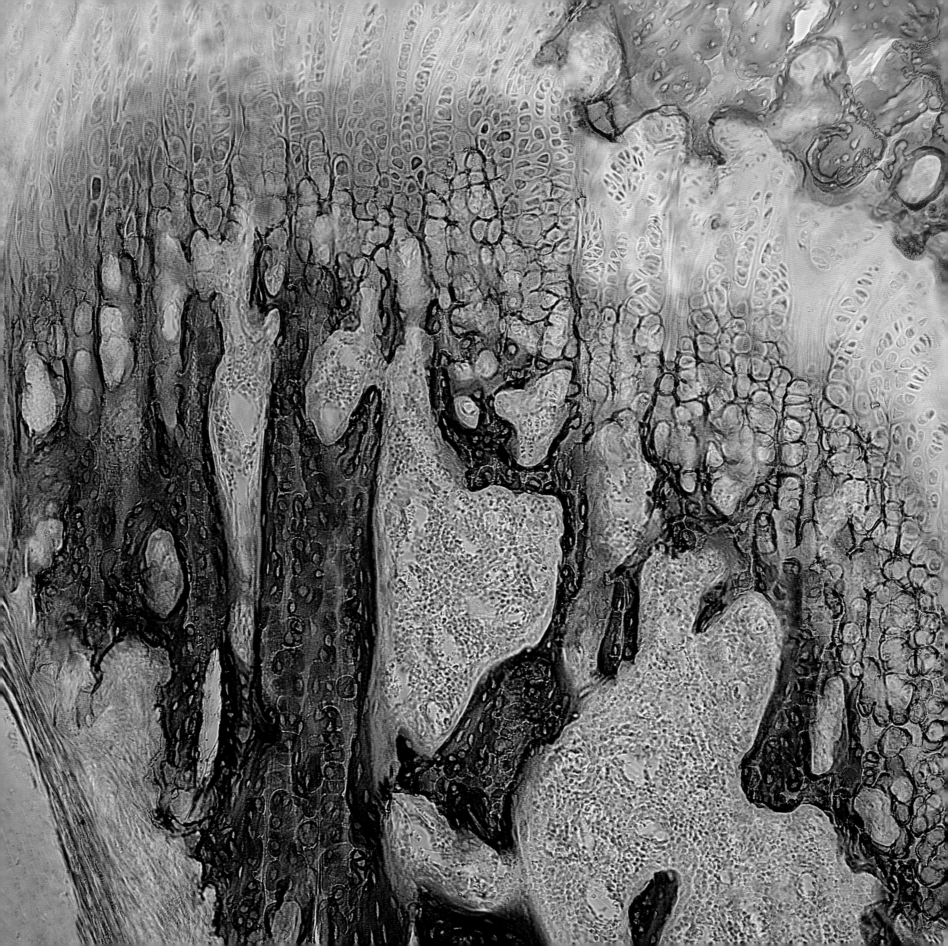

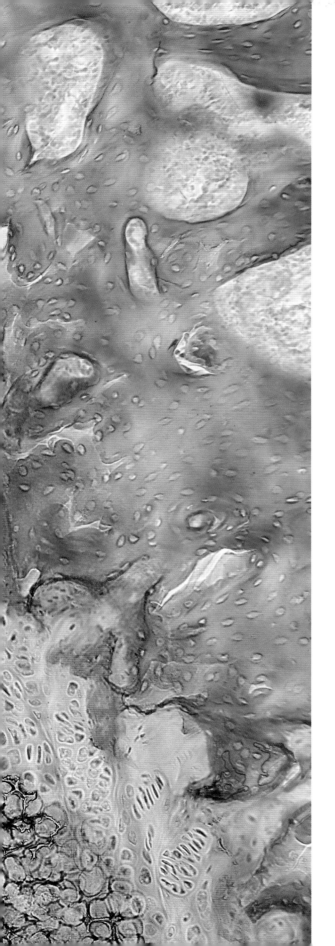

树
未脱钙关节骨与软骨组织磨片，×100，明视野 + 偏振光，2019

Tree
Bone and cartilage, Grounding tissue section, ×100, Light field + polarized light, 2019

花 雨 江 南

Beautiful Rainy Jiangnan

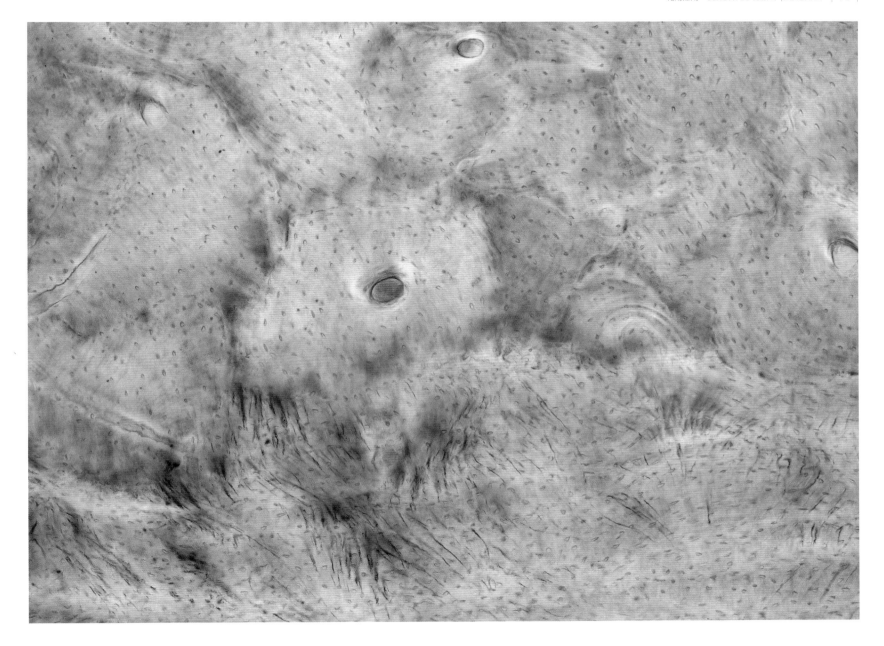

雨后
未脱钙骨组织切片，×100，明视野，2013

After the Rain
Cortical bone, Tissue section, ×100, Light field, 2013

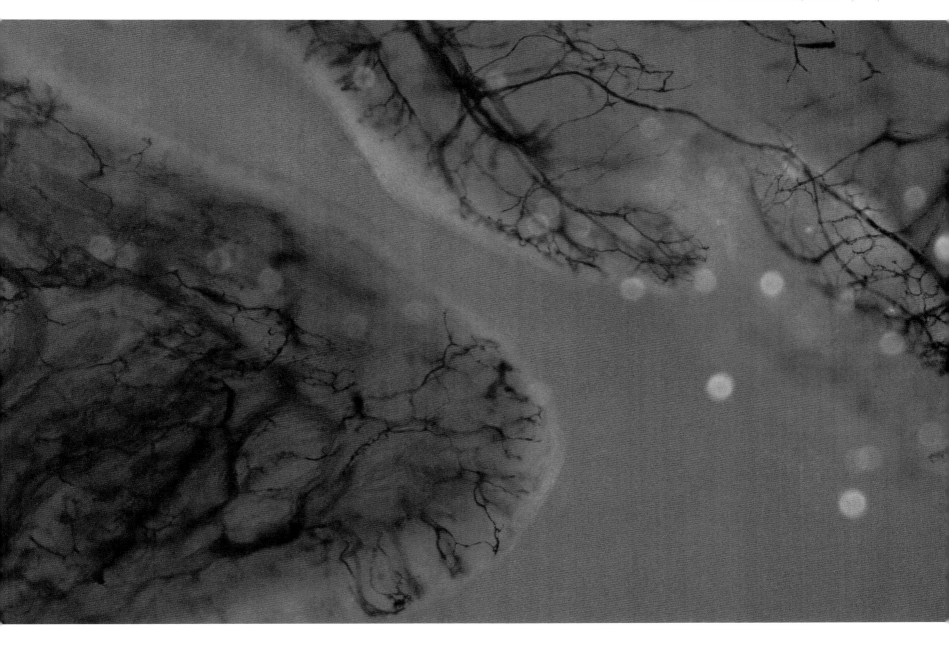

浮萍

灌墨血管和肌肉组织切片，×100，明视野（长时间曝光），2019

The Floating Green

Ink-irrigated blood vessels and muscles, Tissue section, ×100, Light field (long exposure), 2019

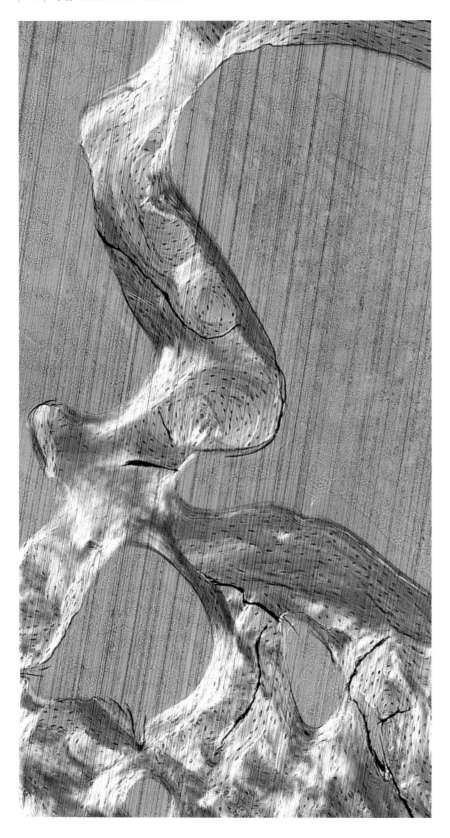

绣屏
未脱钙骨组织磨片，×100，明视野 + 偏振光，2019

Embroidery Screen
Trabecular bone, Grounding section, ×100, Light field +polarized light, 2019

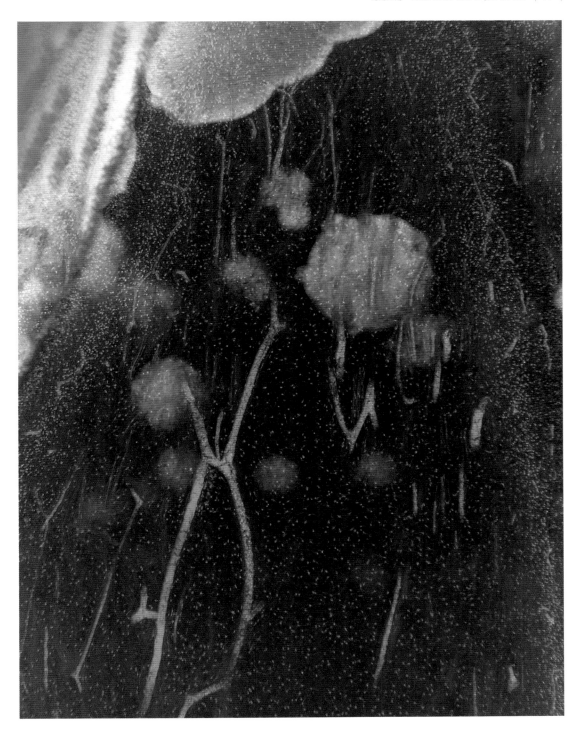

紫雨
牙髓组织切片，×40，荧光，2011

Purple Rain
Deantal pulp, Tissue section, ×40, Fluorescence, 2011

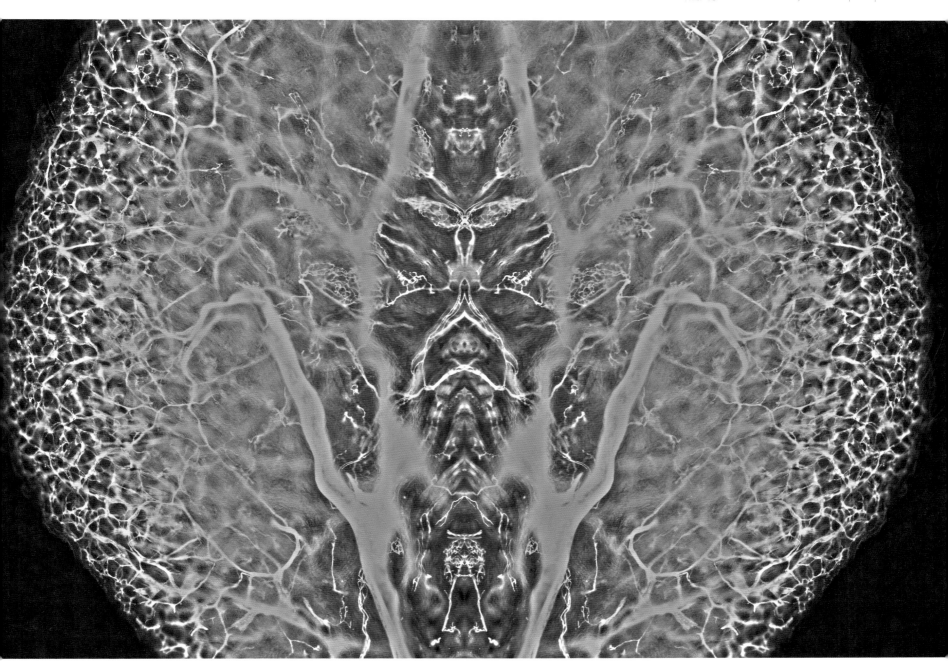

玉树

灌墨血管组织切片的局部镜像，×40，偏振光负像，2014

Tree of Jade

Mirror image of part of ink-irrigated blood vessels tissue section, ×40, Negative image of polarized light, 2014

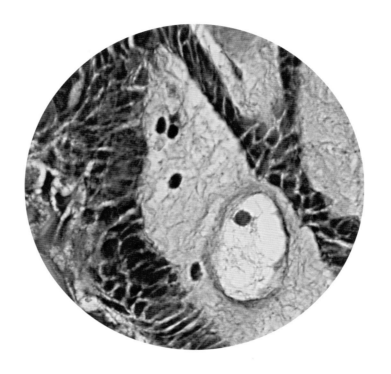

紫藤

牙源性上皮组织切片，×100，明视野，2011

Wisteria

Epithelium, Tissue section, ×100, Light field, 2011

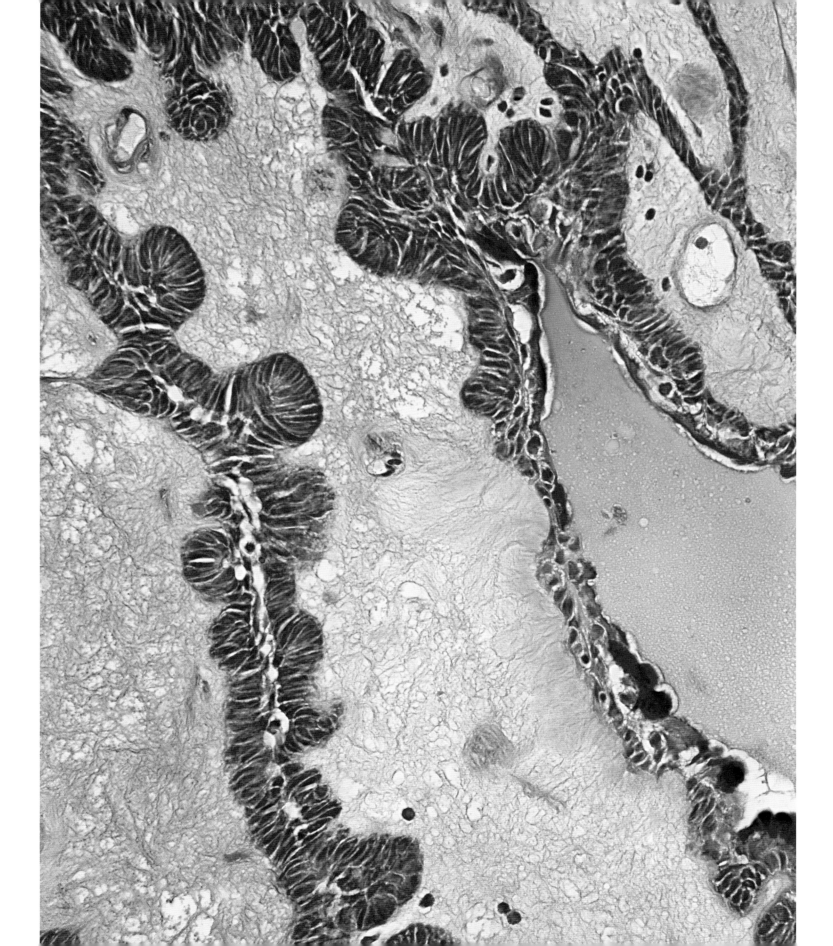

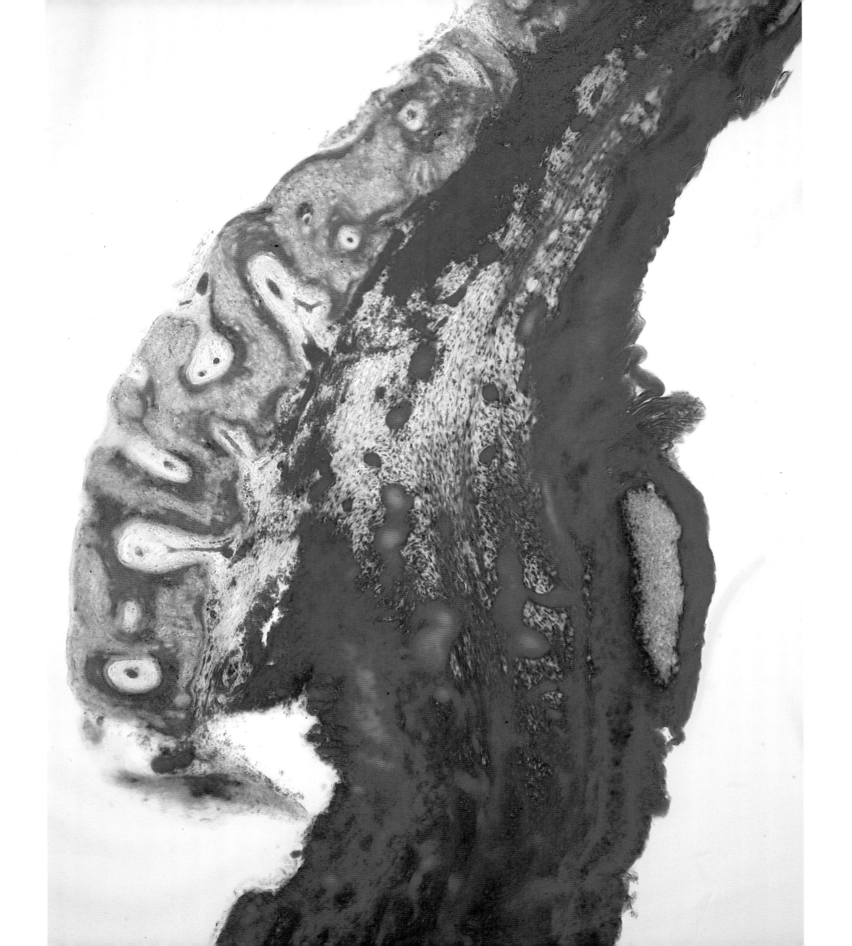

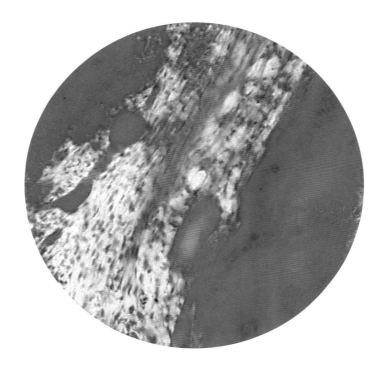

红蘑菇

脱钙骨组织切片，×12.5，明视野，2012

Red Mushroom

Cortical and trabecular bone, Tissue section, ×12.5, Light field, 2012

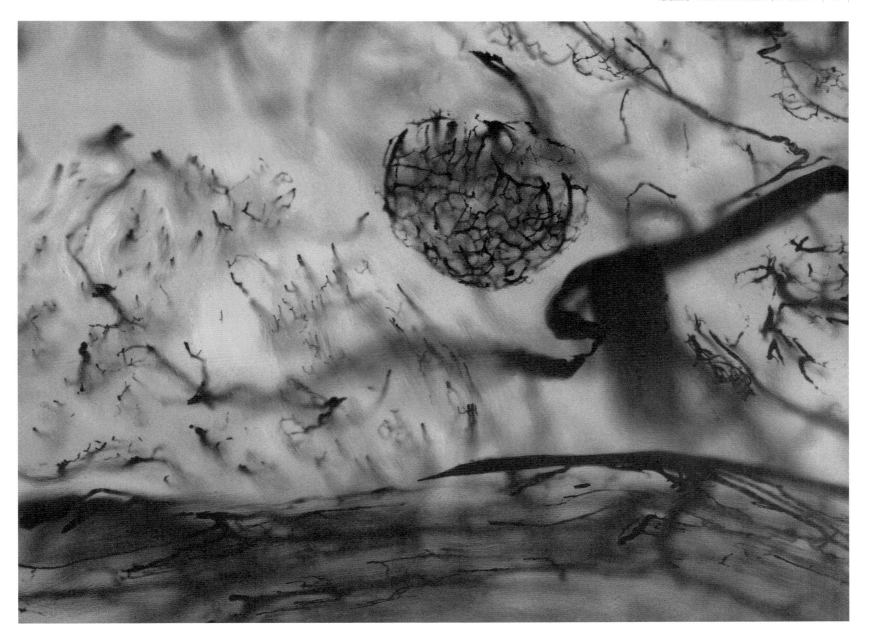

金色果园

灌墨血管组织切片，×40，明视野（长时间曝光），2019

Golden Orchard

Ink-irrigated blood vessels, Tissue section, ×40, Light field (long exposure), 2019

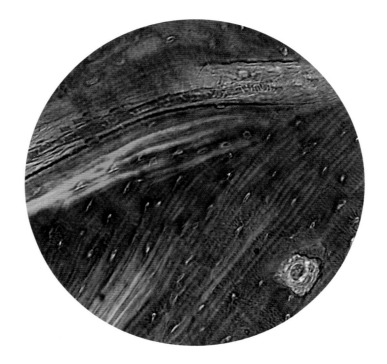

花谷
脱钙骨组织切片，×100，偏振光，2019

Flower Valley
Cortical bone, Tissue section, ×100, Polarized light, 2019

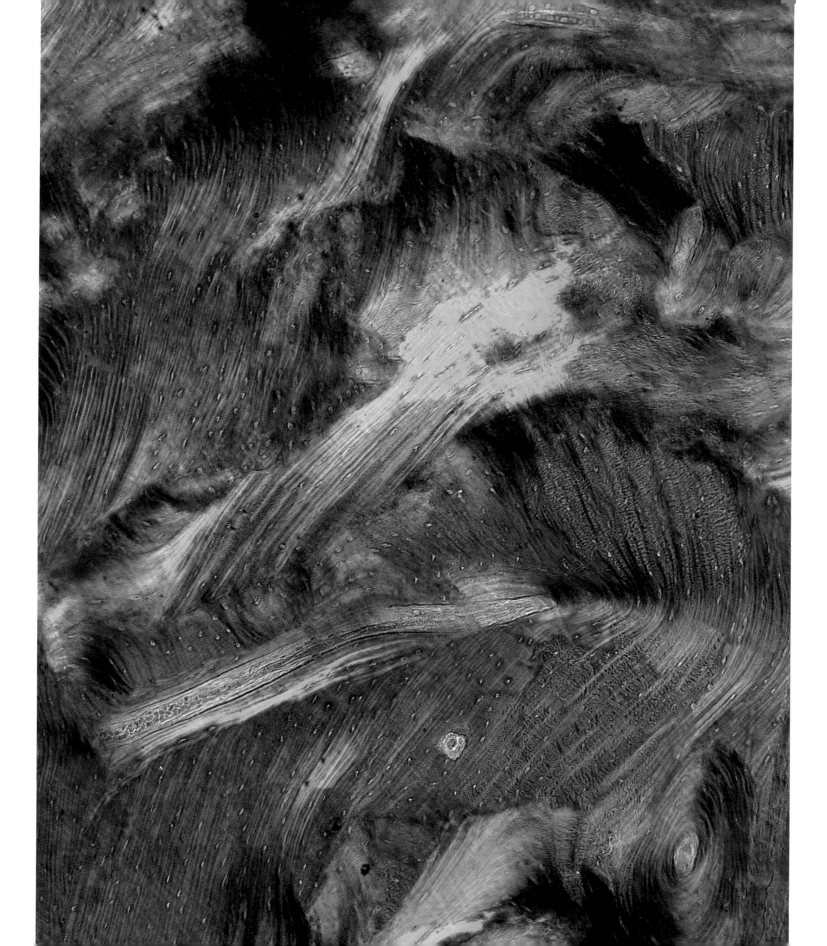

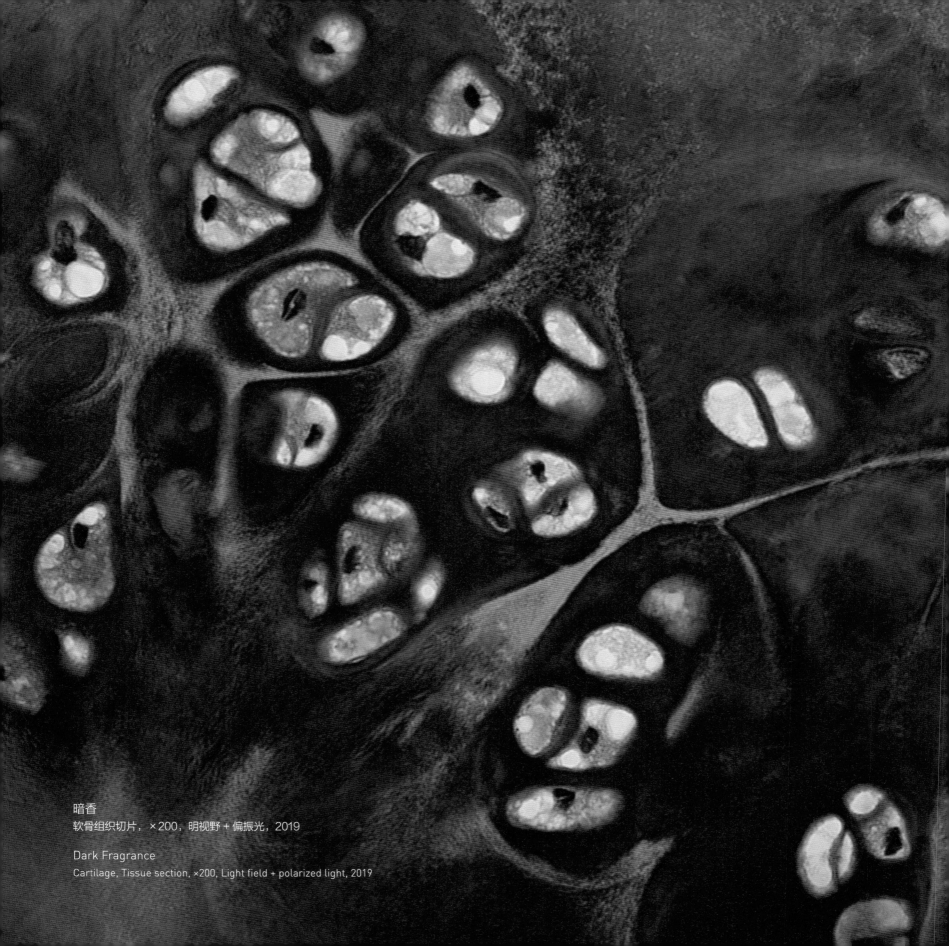

暗香
软骨组织切片，×200，明视野＋偏振光，2019

Dark Fragrance
Cartilage, Tissue section, ×200, Light field + polarized light, 2019

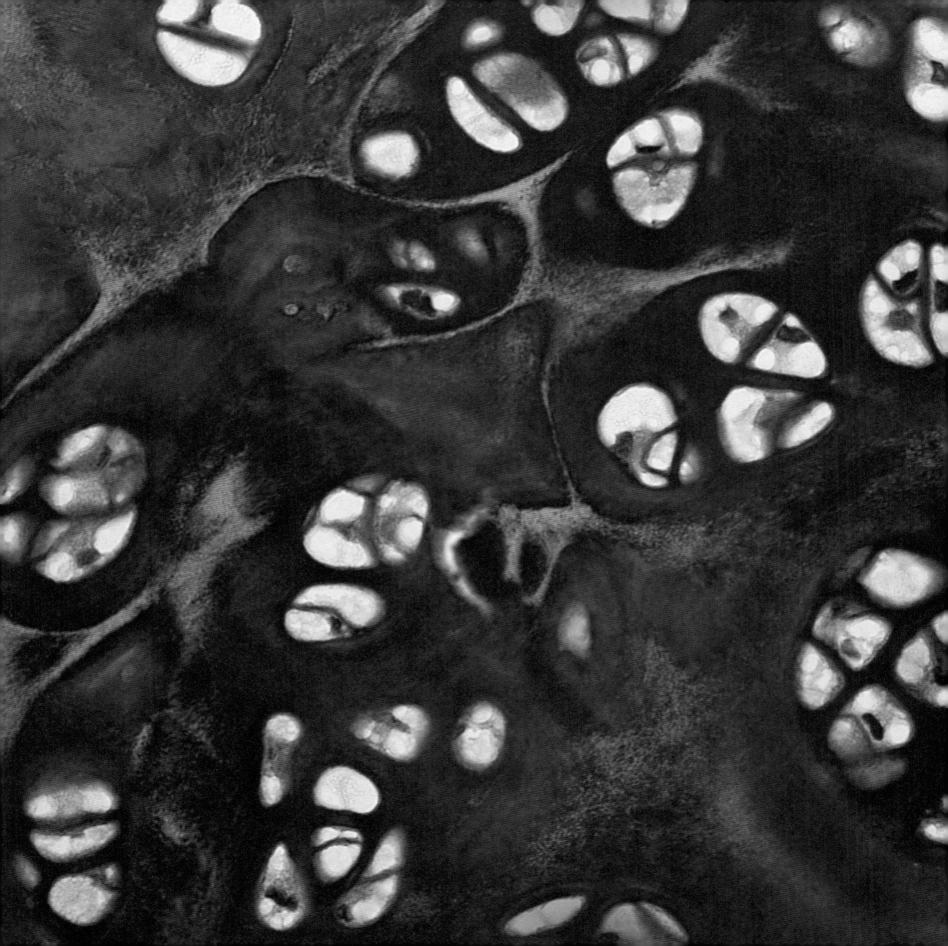

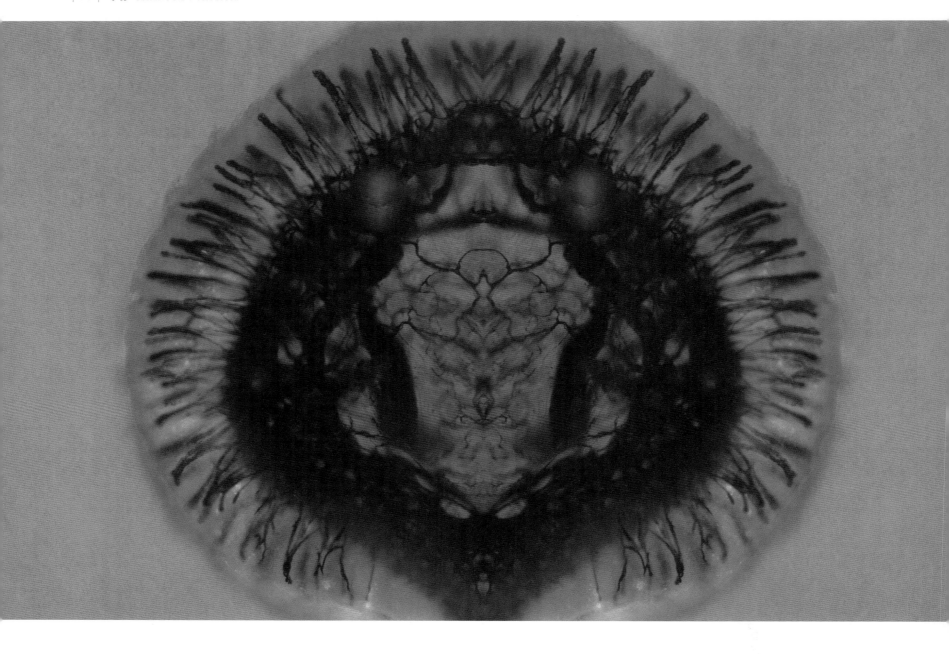

狝猴梦境

灌墨血管组织切片的局部镜像，×100，明视野（长时间曝光），2019

Kiwi Dream

Mirror image of part of ink-irrigated blood vessels, Tissue section, ×100, Light field (long exposure), 2019

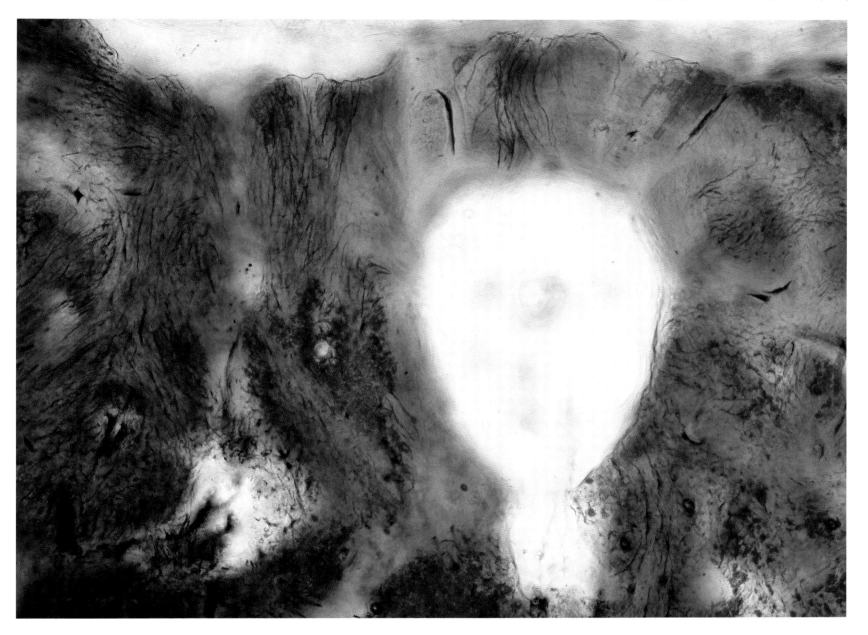

小桥旁边

未脱钙骨组织磨片，×40，明视野，2013

By the Small Bridge

Cortical bone, Grounding tissue section, ×40, Light field, 2013

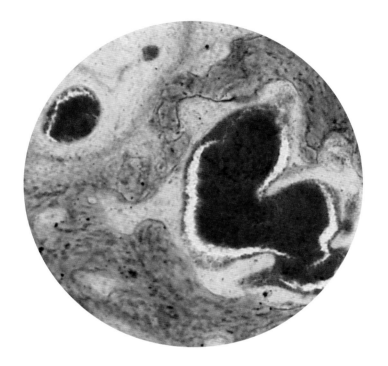

青花

脱钙鼻甲组织切片，×12.5，明视野，2011

Blue and White Porcelain

Turbinate tissue, Tissue section, ×12.5, Light field, 2011

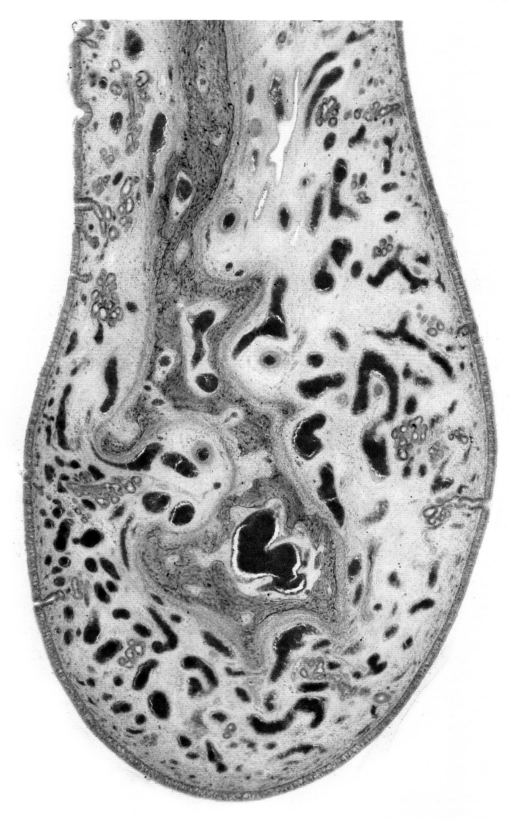

林间萤火

未脱钙骨组织及周围软组织磨片，×40，偏振光，2019

Fireflies in the Woods

Soft tissues surrounding the bone, Grounding section, ×40, Polarized light, 2019

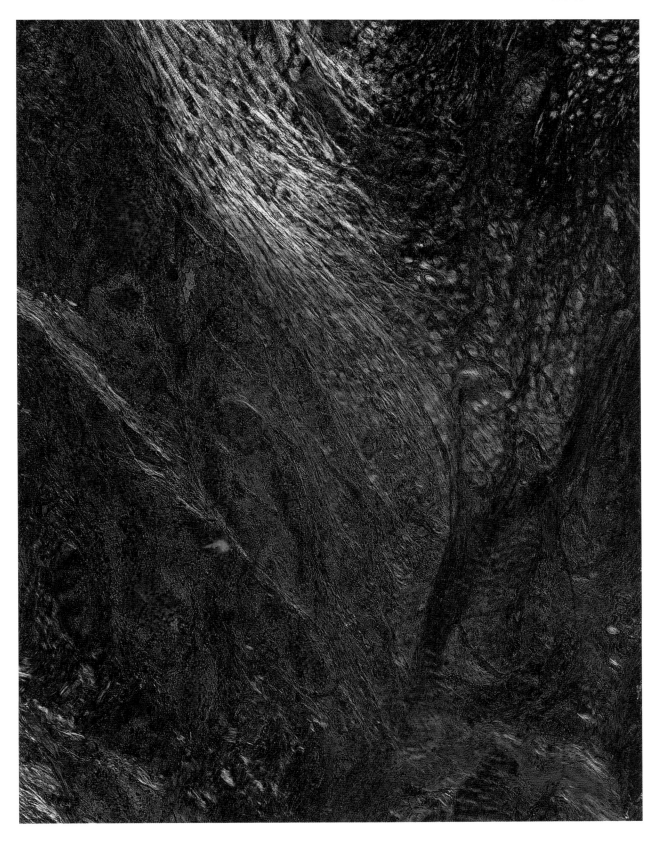

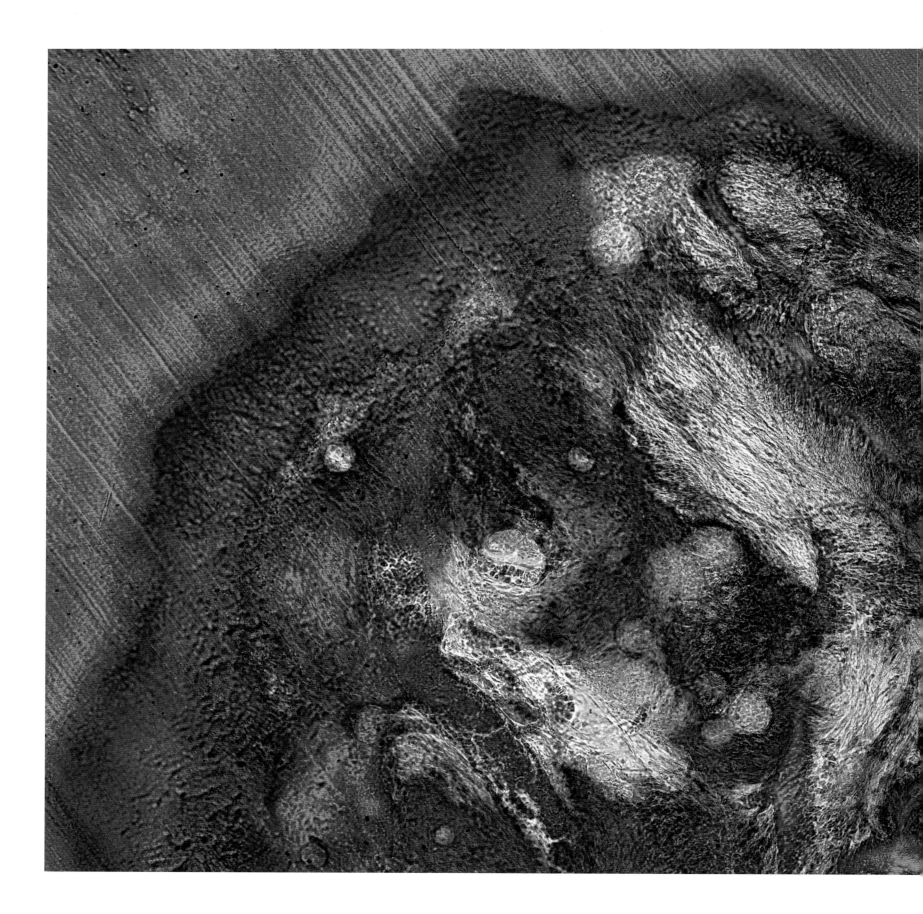

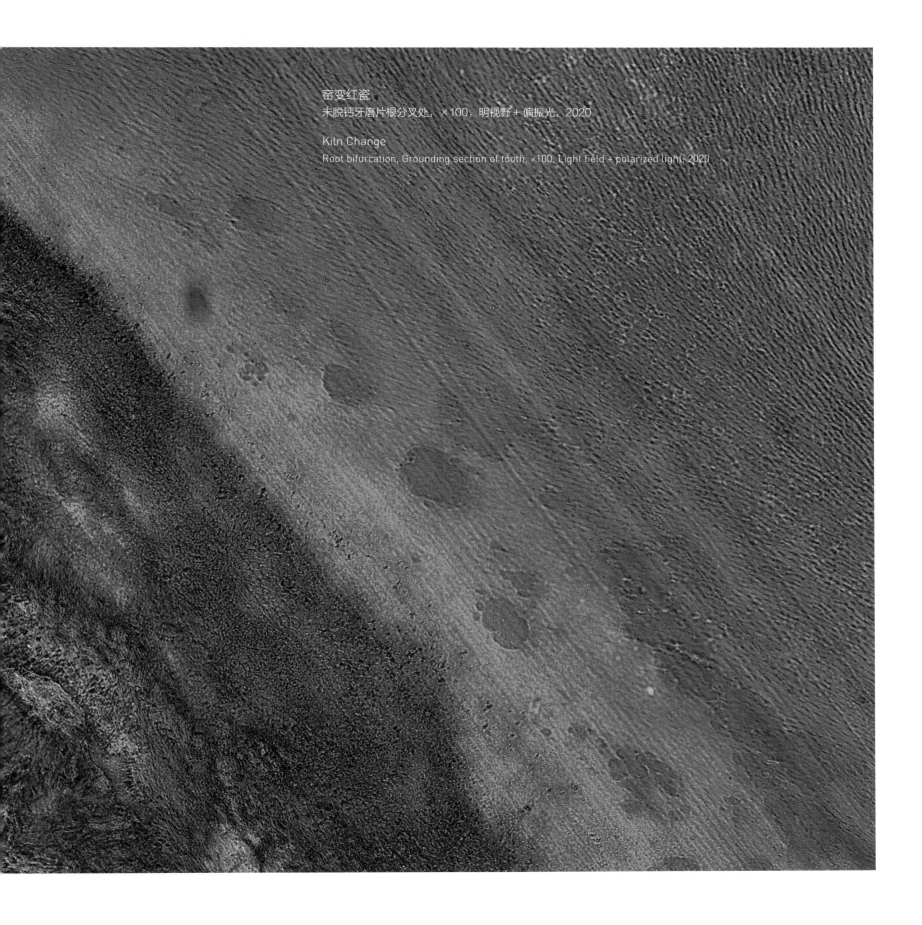

窑变红瓷
未脱钙牙磨片根分叉处，×100；明视野＋偏振光，2020

Kiln Change
Root bifurcation, Grounding section of tooth, ×100, Light field + polarized light, 2020

一束玫瑰
未脱钙骨组织磨片，×100，偏振光，2019

A Bunch of Roses
Cortical bone, Grounding section, ×100, Polarized light, 2019

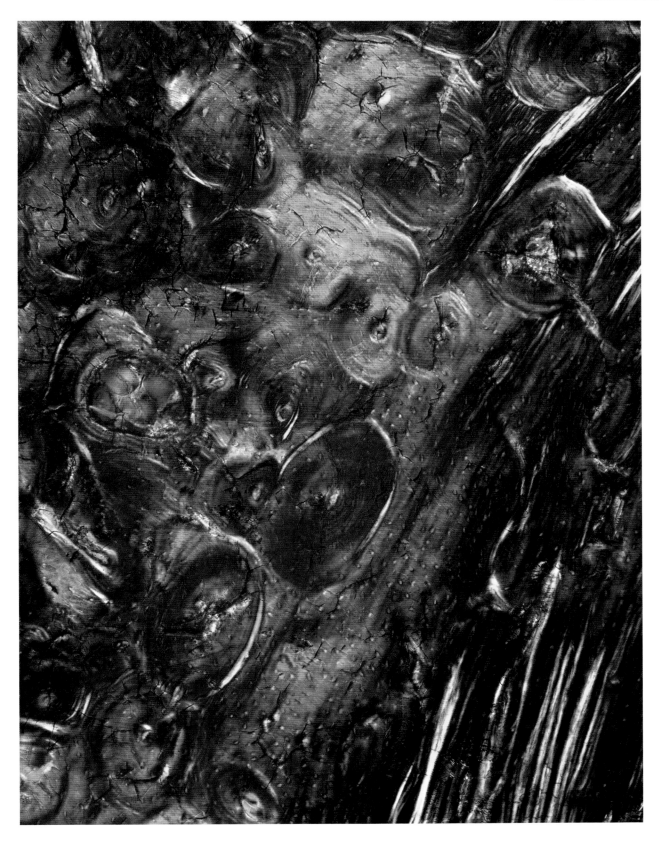

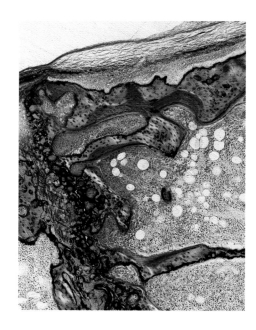

长袖

未脱钙骨组织磨片，×100，明视野＋偏振光，2019

Long Sleeve

Trabecular bone, Grounding section, ×100, Light field + polarized light, 2019

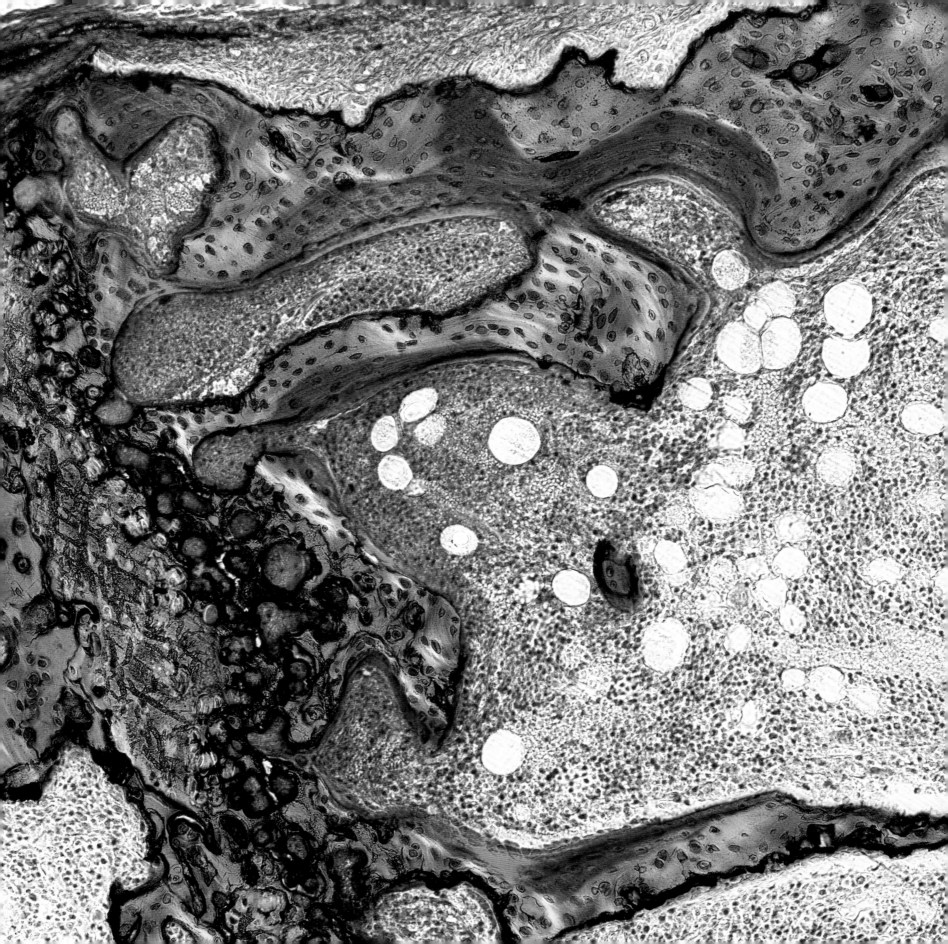

④

时 空 寻 迹

SEARCHING FOR THE TIME AND SPACE

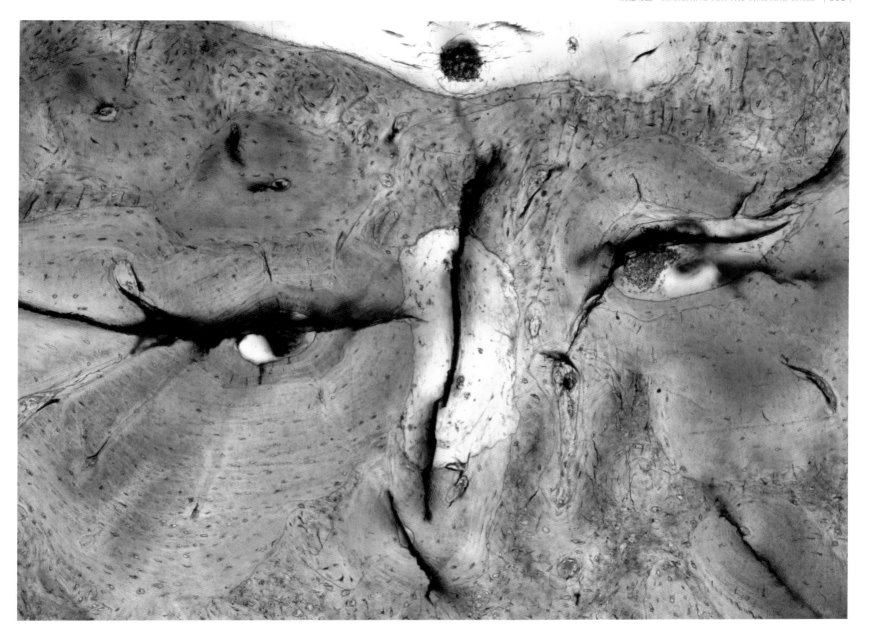

石佛
未脱钙骨组织硬组织切片，×100，明视野，2013

Stone Buddha
Cortical bone, Grounding tissue section, ×100, Light field, 2013

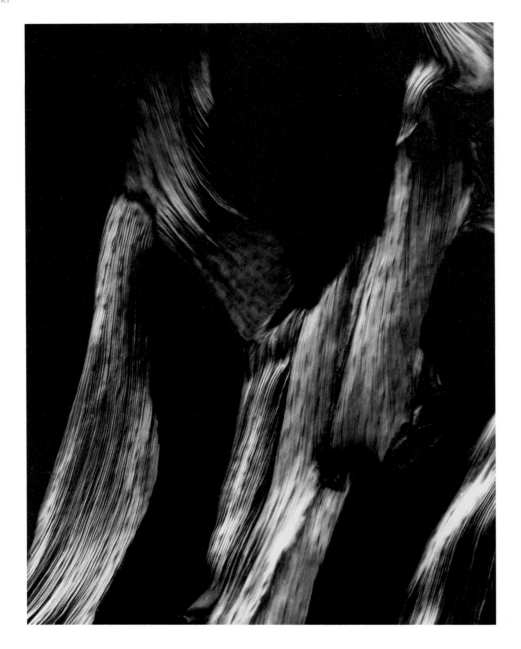

熔岩

脱钙骨组织切片，×100，偏振光，2013

Lava

Trabecular bone, Tissue section, ×100, Polarized light, 2013

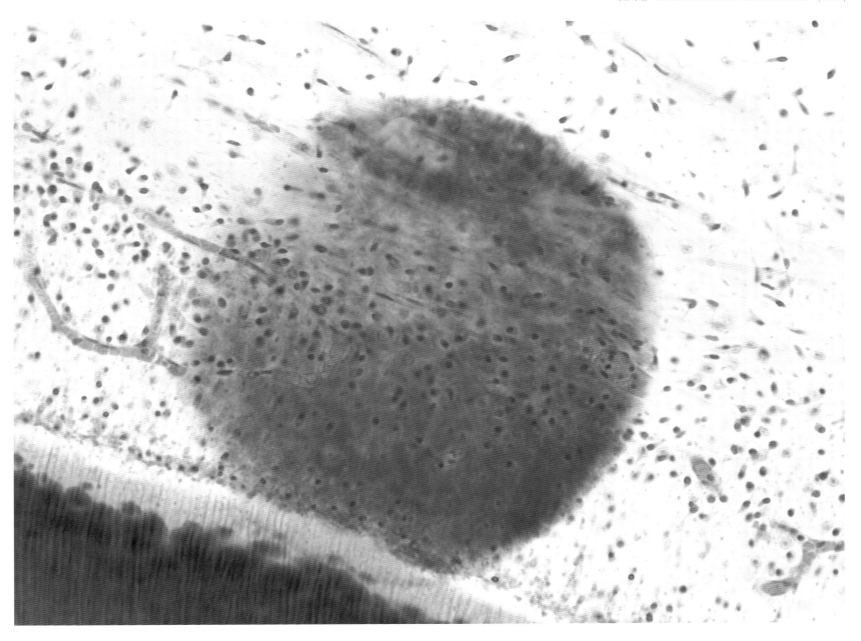

飞石

牙髓及牙本质组织切片，×100，明视野，2011

Flying Stone

Pulp stone and dentin, Tissue section, ×100, Light field, 2011

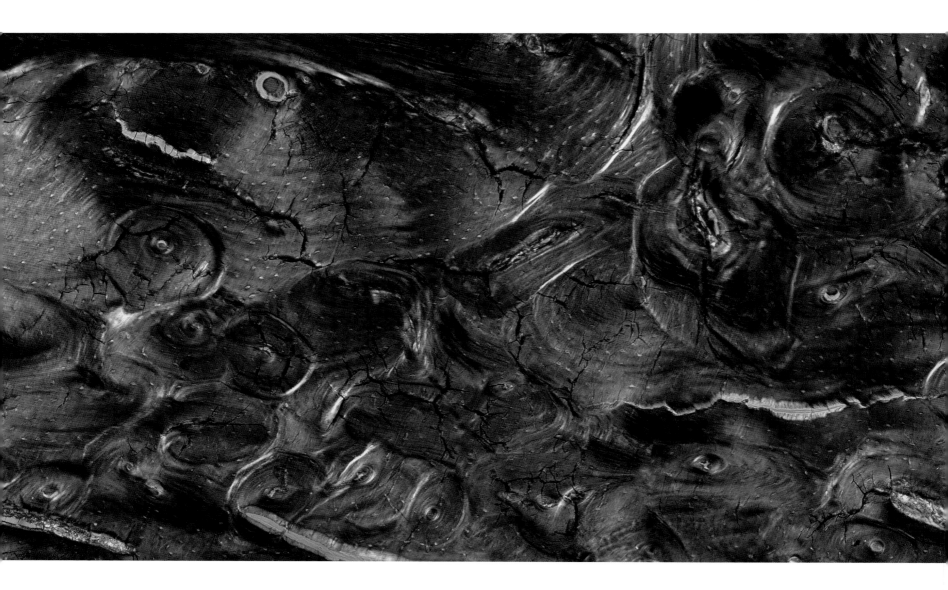

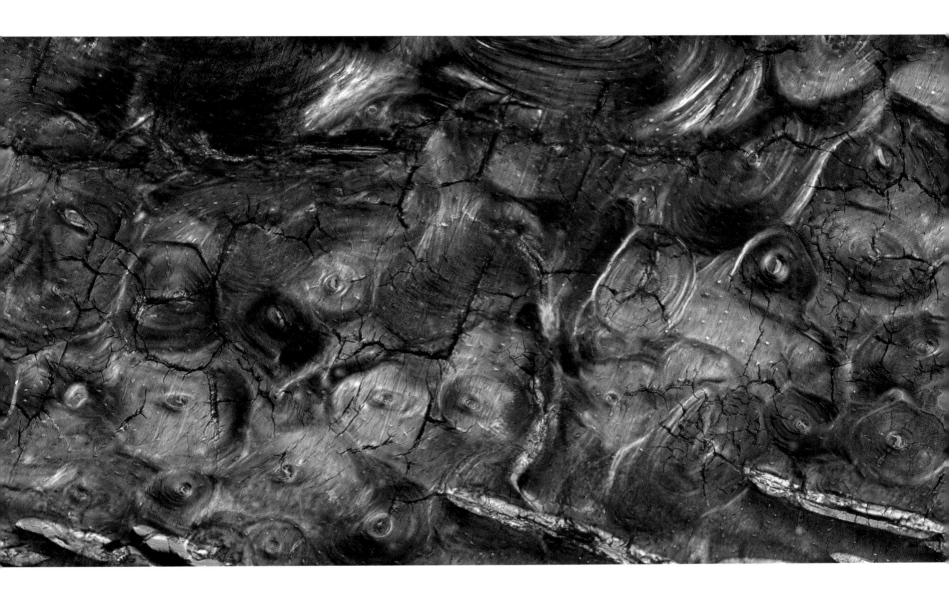

起皱的风景

未脱钙骨组织磨片，×100，偏振光，2019

Wrinkled Scenery

Cortical bone, Grounding tissue section, ×100, Polarized light, 2019

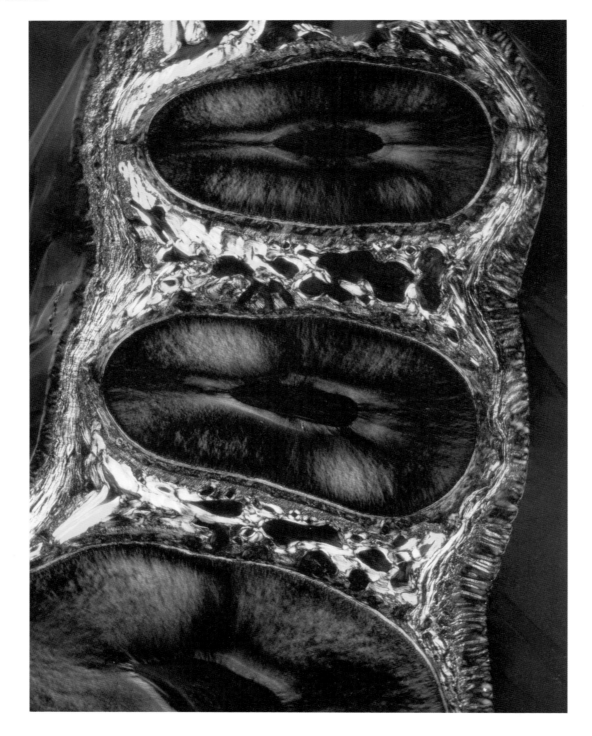

镶钻

牙槽骨、牙根及牙龈组织联合切片，×12.5，偏振光，2013

Diamond

Tooth root and periodontium, Combined section of tooth and jaw, ×12.5, Polarized light, 2013

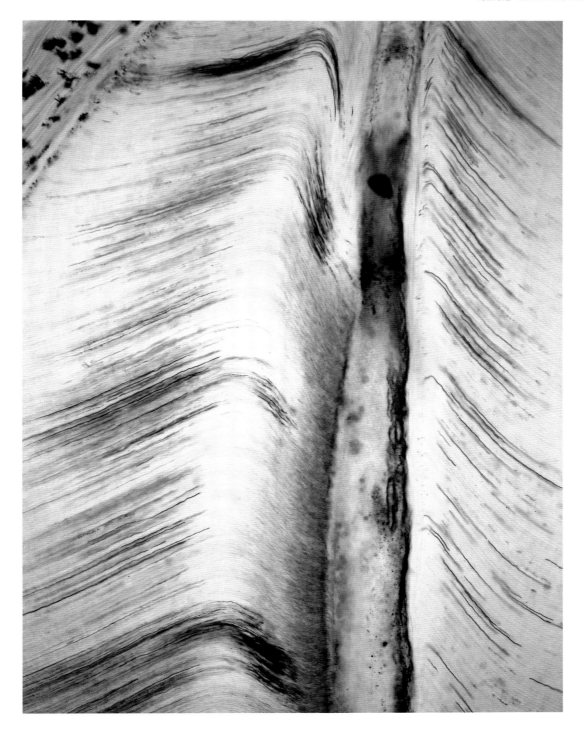

幽谷

未脱钙牙齿根部磨片，×12.5，明视野，2011

Canyon

Tooth root with canal, Grounding section, ×12.5, Light field, 2011

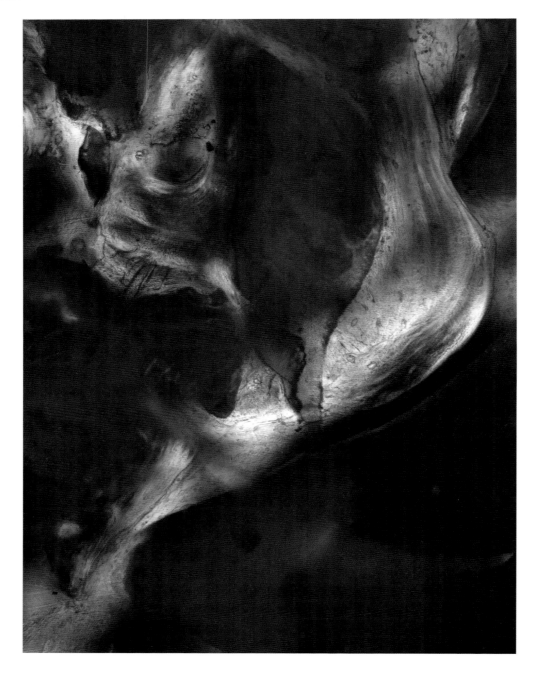

私密
未脱钙骨组织磨片，×100，偏振光，2013

Private Secret
Trabecular bone, Grounding tissue section, ×100, Polarized light, 2013

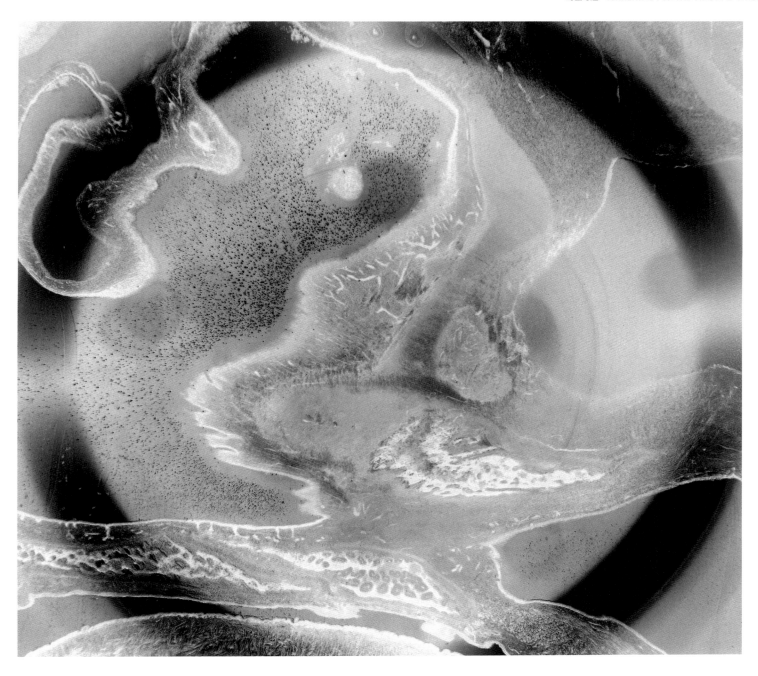

幻影
鼻腔黏膜上皮组织切片，×12.5，错用聚光镜后的意外影像，2013

Phantom
Nosal mucosa, Tissue section, ×12.5, Light field with wrong use of condenser lens, 2013

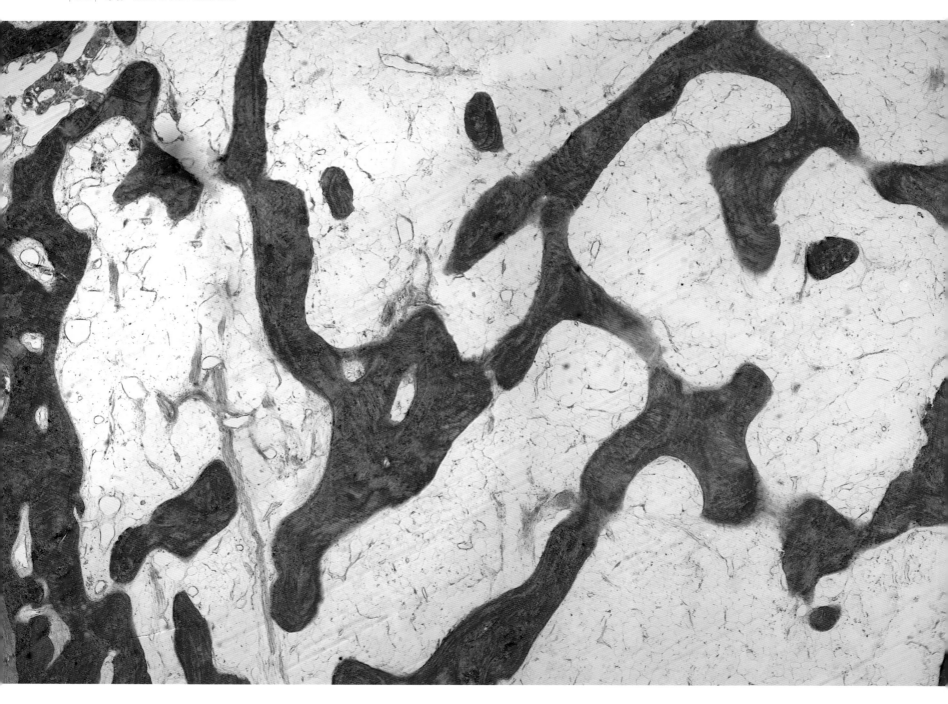

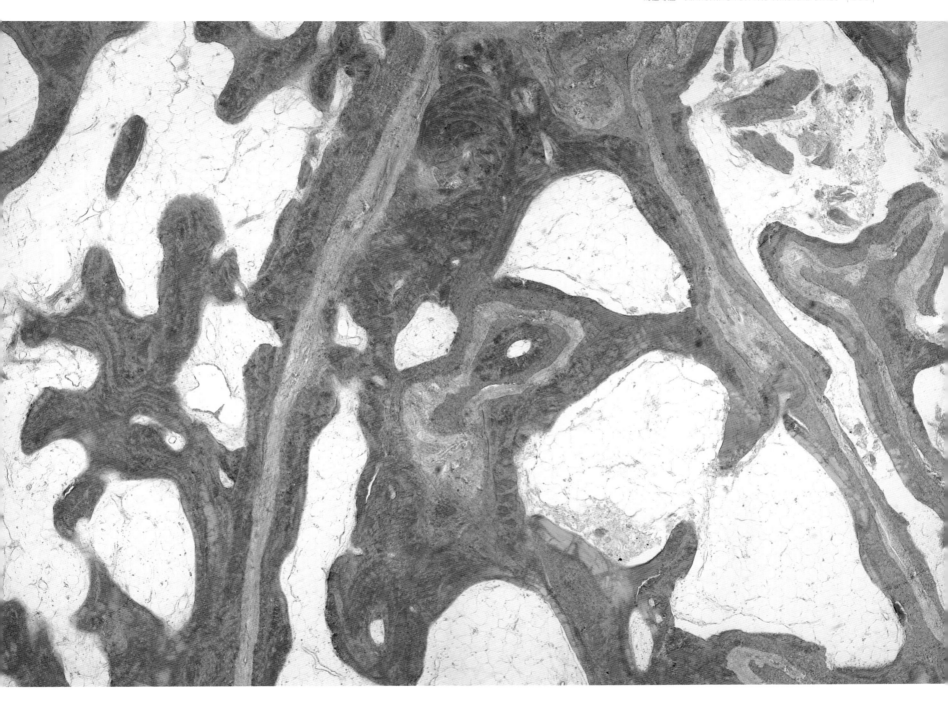

图腾

脱钙骨组织切片，×40，明视野＋偏振光，2016

Totem

Trabecular bone, Tissue section, ×40, Light field+polarized light, 2016

甲骨文 No.1

脱钙骨组织切片，×40，明视野，2015

Oracle No.1

Trabecular bone, Tissue section, ×40, Light field, 2015

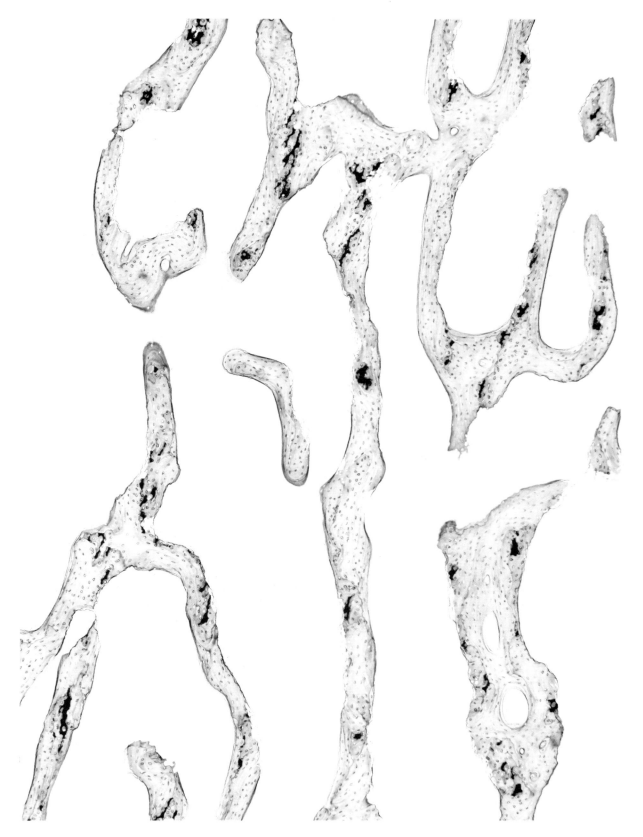

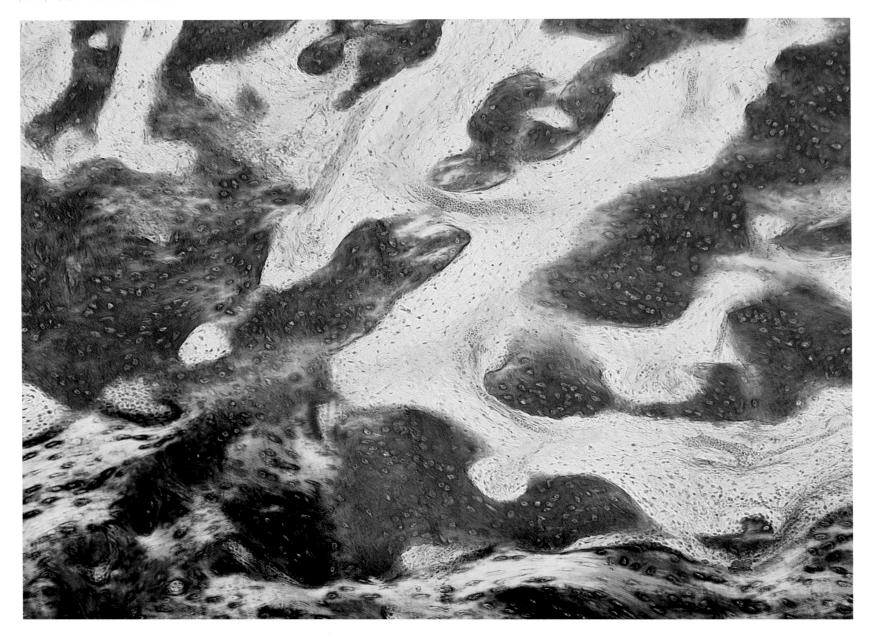

飞天

脱钙骨组织切片，×100，明视野 + 偏振光，2019

Flying

Trabecular bone, Tissue section, ×100, Light field+polarized light, 2019

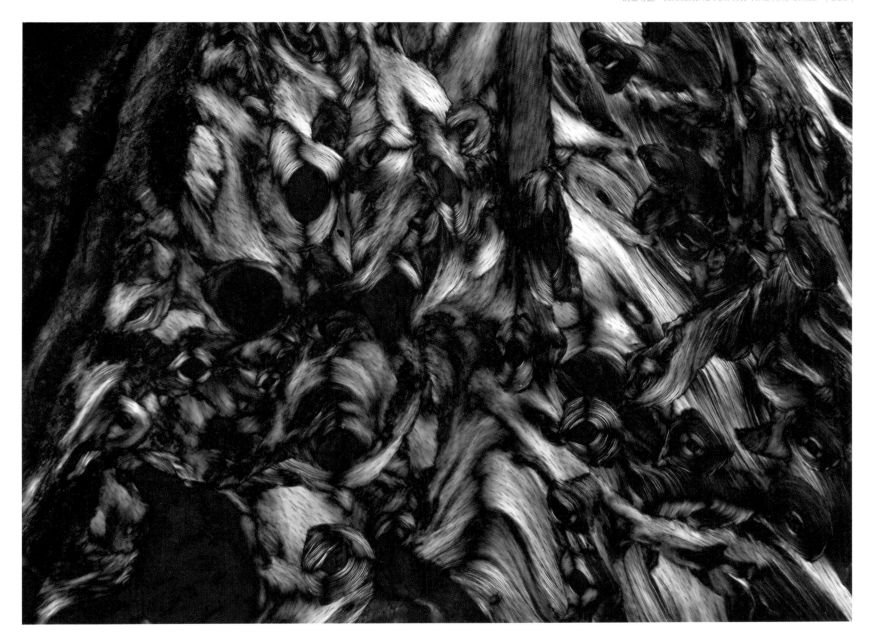

凝固的时间
脱钙骨组织切片，×40，偏振光，2015

Time of Solidification
Cortical bone, Tissue section, ×40, Polarized light, 2015

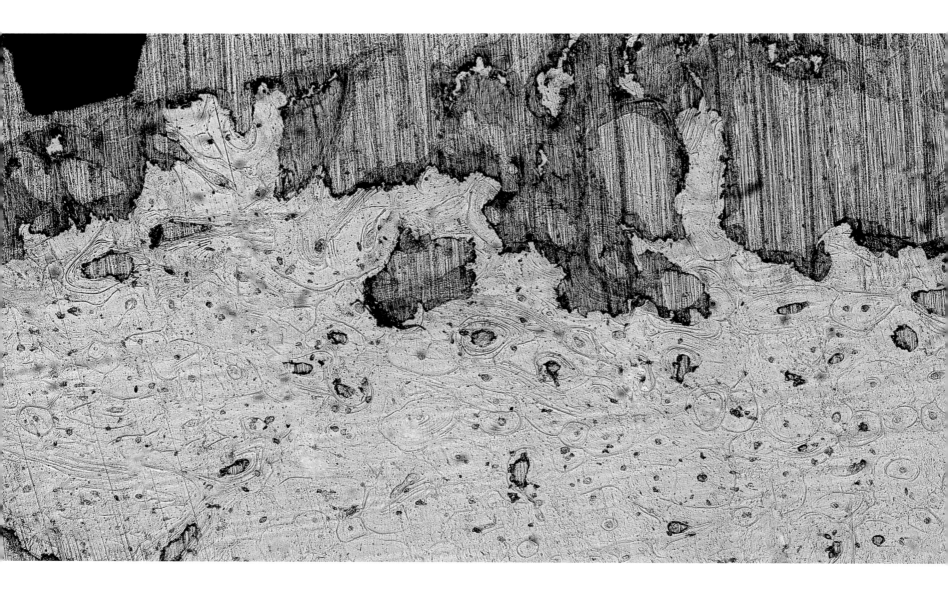

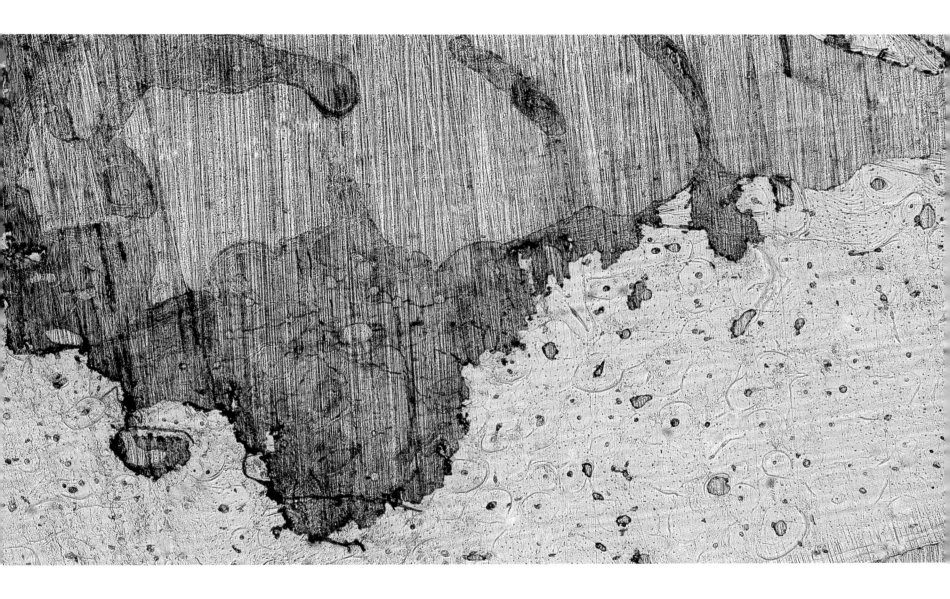

遗落手稿

未脱钙骨组织磨片局部脱落，×40，明视野 + 偏振光，2019

Lost Script

Cortical bone, Grounding tissue section, ×40, Light field + polarized light, 2019

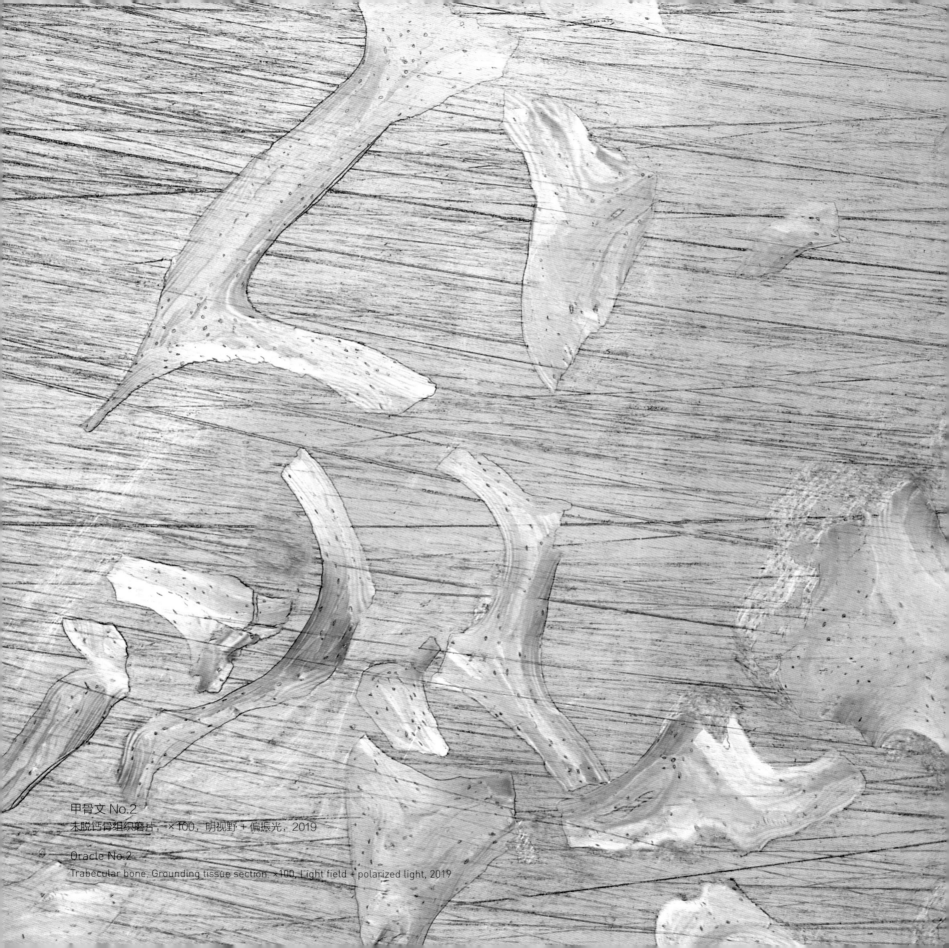

甲骨文 No.2

未脱钙骨组织磨片，×100，明视野＋偏振光，2019

Oracle No.2

Trabecular bone. Grounding tissue section. ×100, Light field + polarized light, 2019

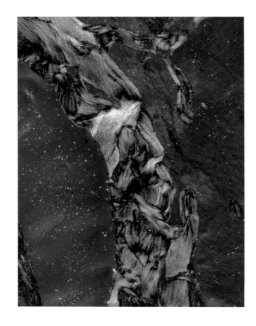

不朽

脱钙骨组织切片，×40，偏振光，2013

Immortality

Trabecular bone, Tissue section, ×40, Polarized light, 2013

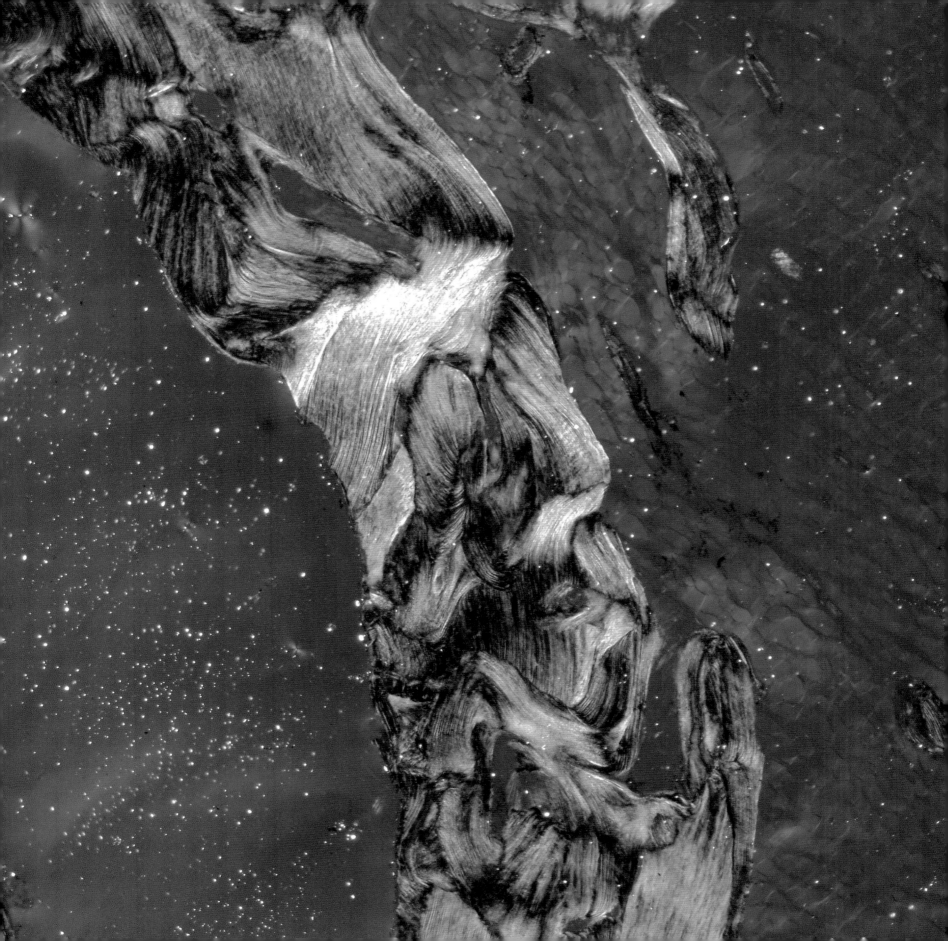

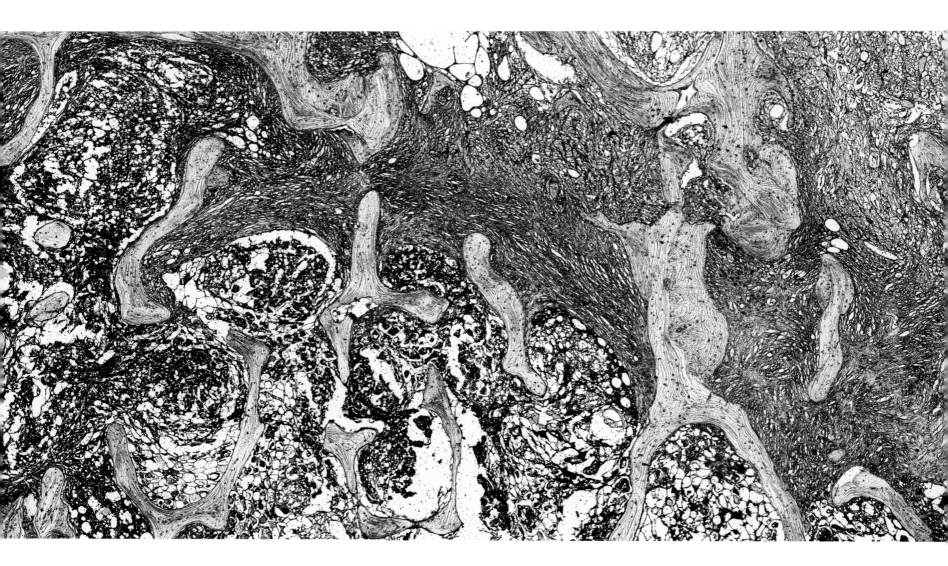

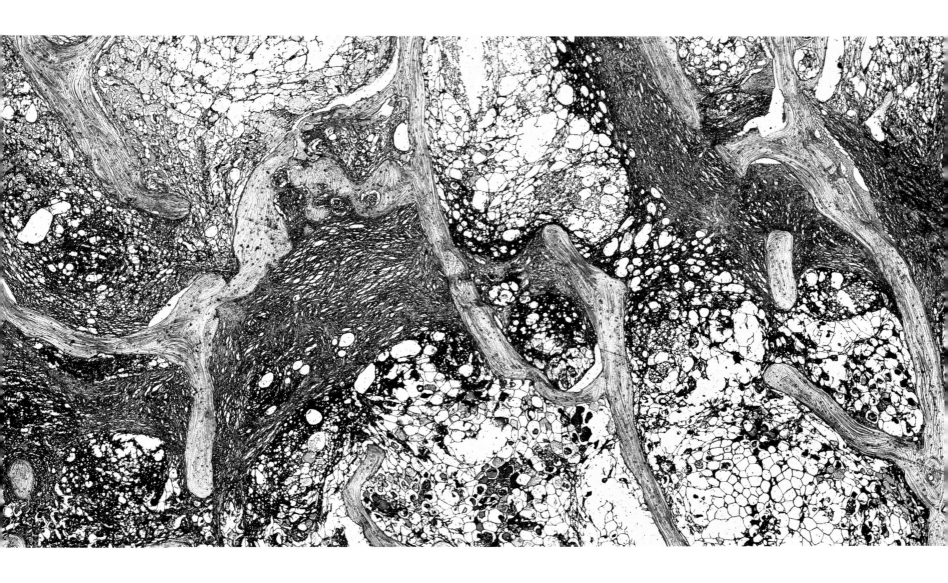

甲骨文 No.3

未脱钙骨组织磨片，×40，明视野 + 偏振光，2019

Oracle No.3

Trabecular bone, Grounding tissue section, ×40, Light field + polarized light, 2019

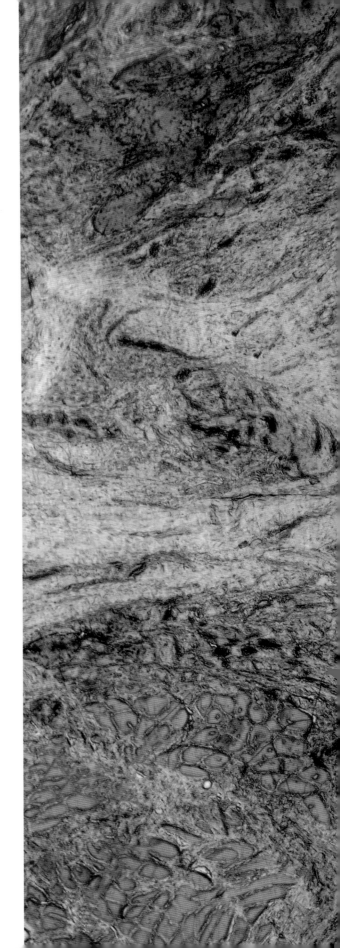

老地图
未脱钙骨及周围软组织磨片，×40，明视野 + 偏振光，2019

Old Map
Bone and surrounding soft tissues, Grounding tissue section, ×40, Light field + polarized light, 2019

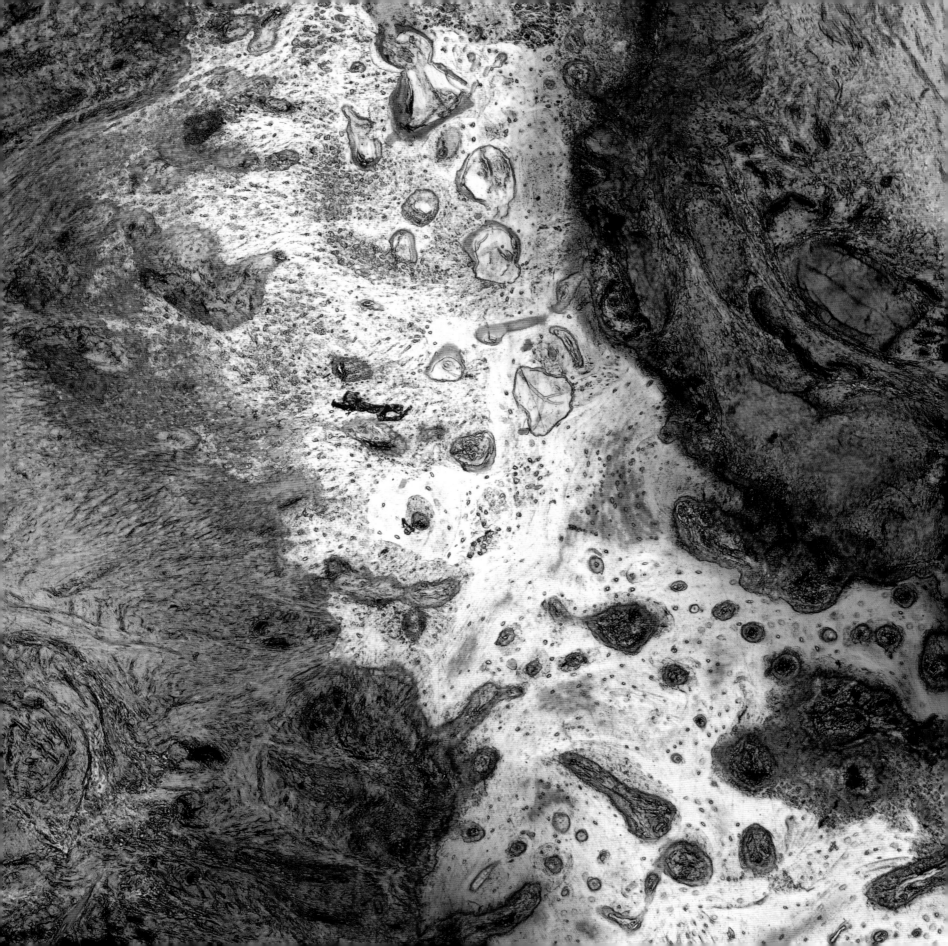

⑤

万 物 并 生

HARMONIZED UNIVERSE

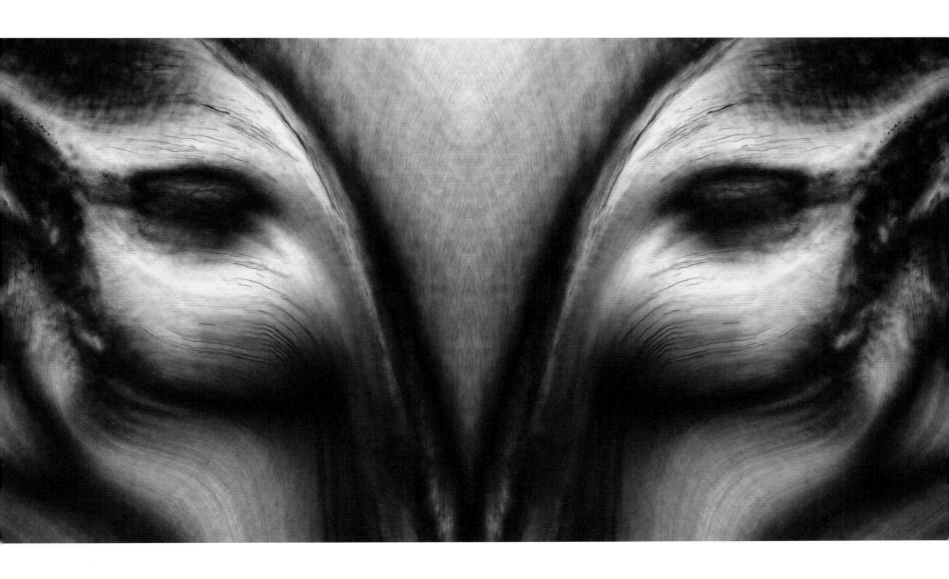

狐仙
未脱钙牙齿磨片根部牙本质的局部镜像，×100，偏振光，2014

Fox Fairy
Mirror image of part of root dentin, Grounding section, ×100, Polarized light, 2014

太极

发育中的软骨、肌肉和血管组织切片，×40，明视野，2013

Tai Chi

Cartiage and muscle, Tissue section, ×40, Light field, 2013

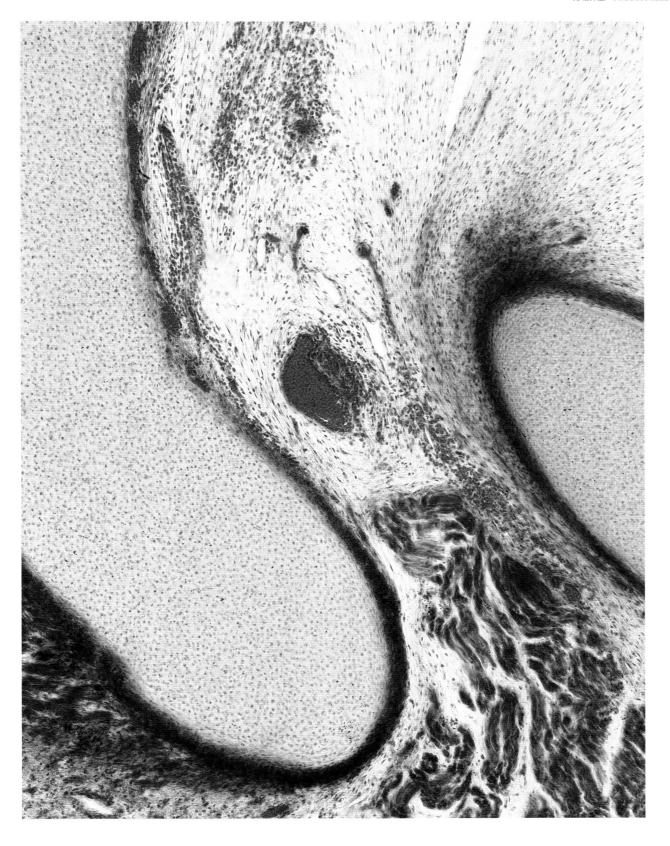

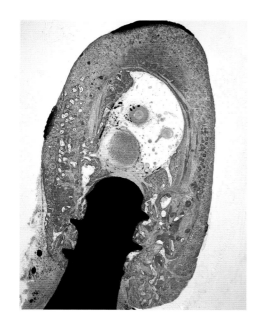

植体的梦想 No.9
未脱钙骨组织与种植体磨片，×12.5，明视野，2019

Dream of Implant No.9
Implant with surrounding bone, Grounding tissue section, ×12.5, Light field, 2019

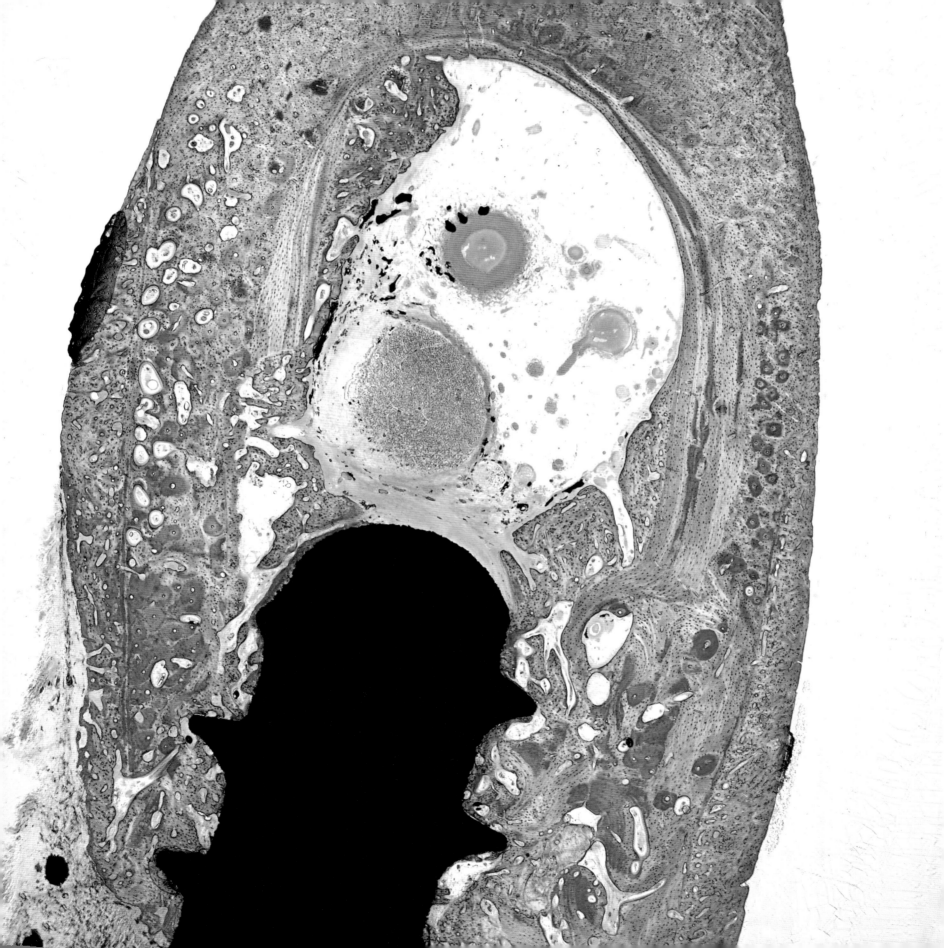

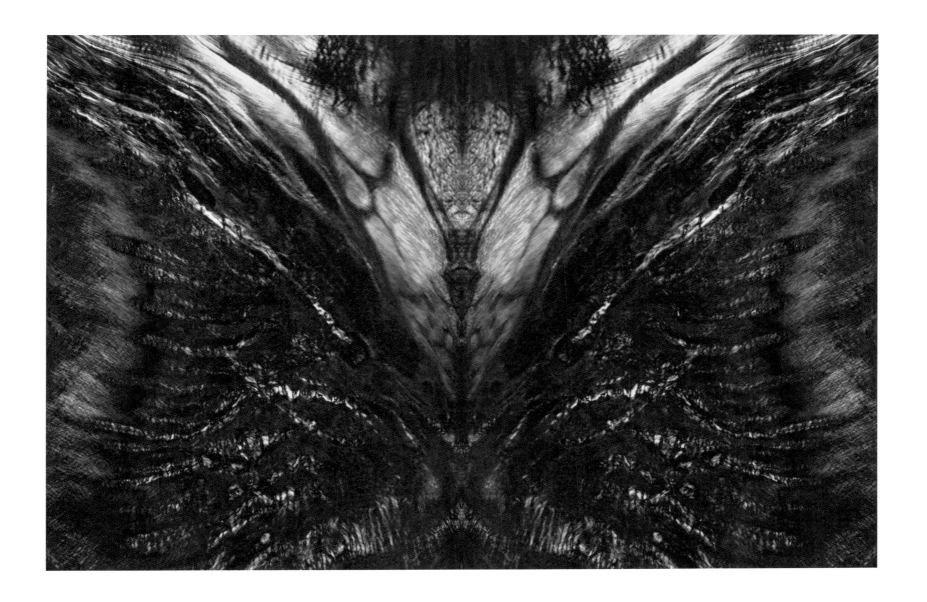

化蝶
牙龈组织切片的局部镜像，×100，偏振光，2014

Butterfly
Mirror image of part of gingival tissue section, ×100, Polarized light, 2014

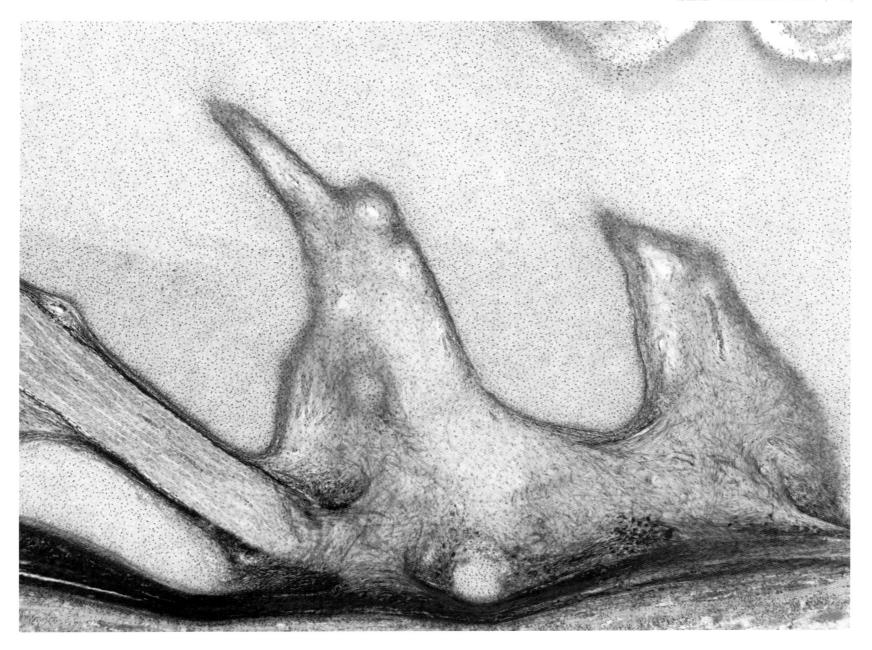

啼鸟
发育中的软骨组织切片，×12.5，明视野，2017

Singing Birds
Developing cartilage, Tissue section, ×12.5, Light field, 2017

俯瞰鸟岛
脱钙骨组织切片和封片胶，×12.5，偏振光，2017

Overlooking the Bird Island
Trabecular bone and sealing glue, Tissue section, ×12.5, Polarized light, 2017

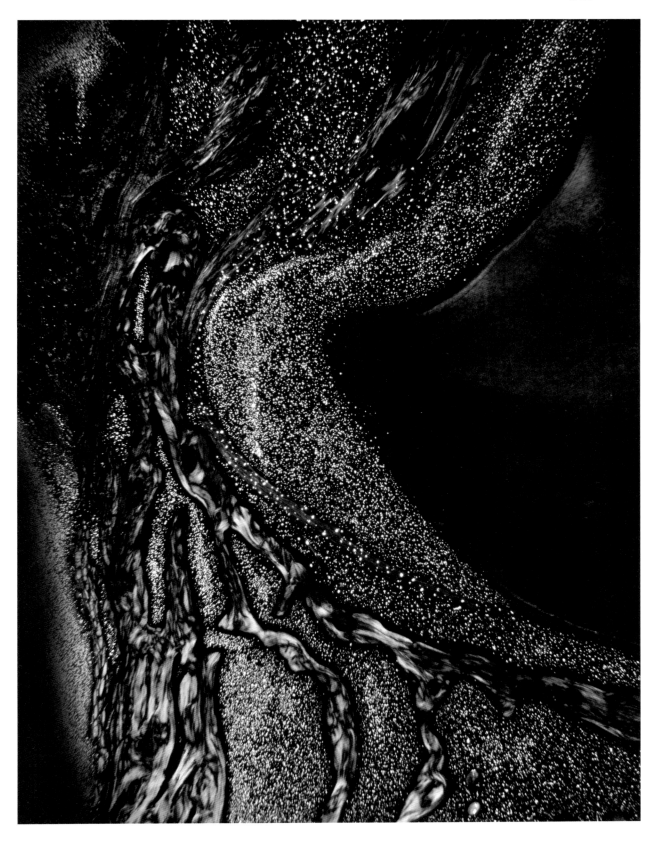

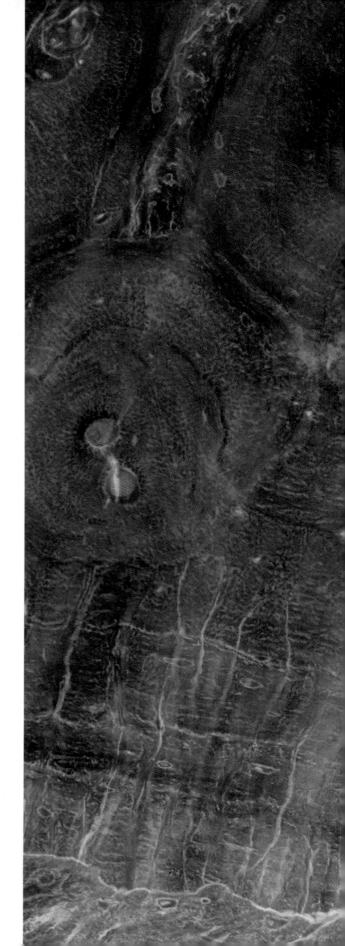

开屏
未脱钙骨组织磨片，×100，偏振光，2013

Dream of Peacock
Cortical bone, Grounding section, ×100, Polarized light, 2013

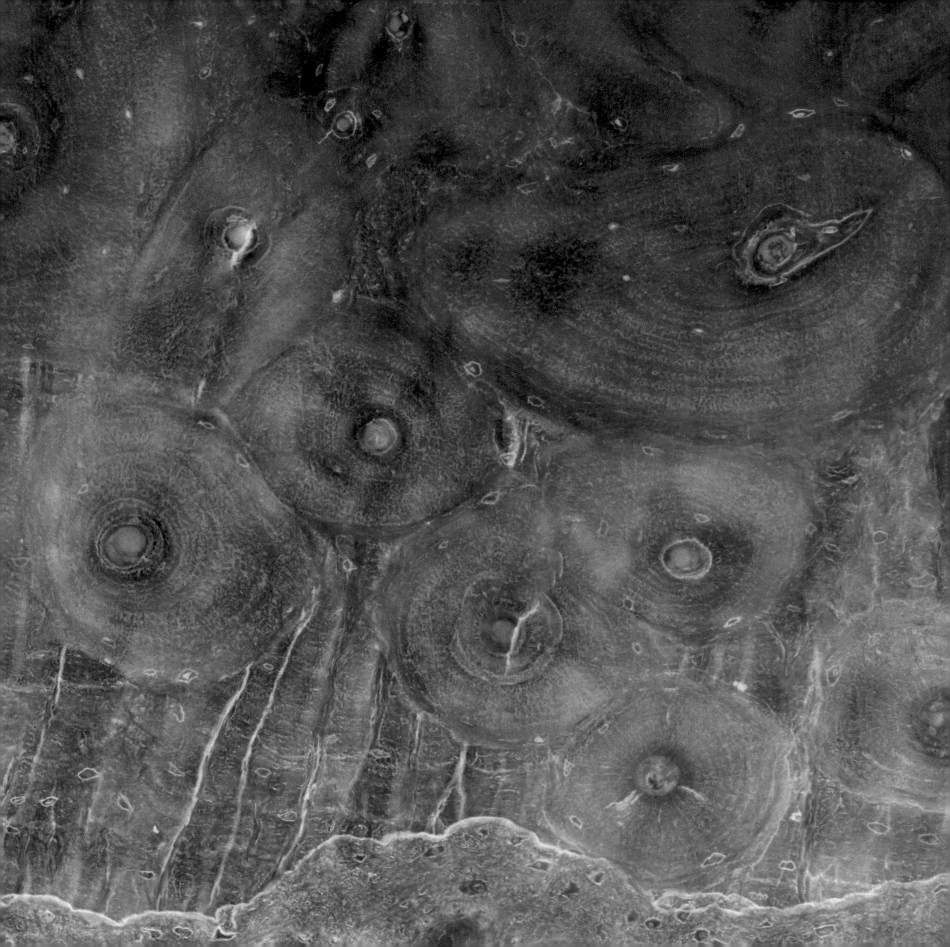

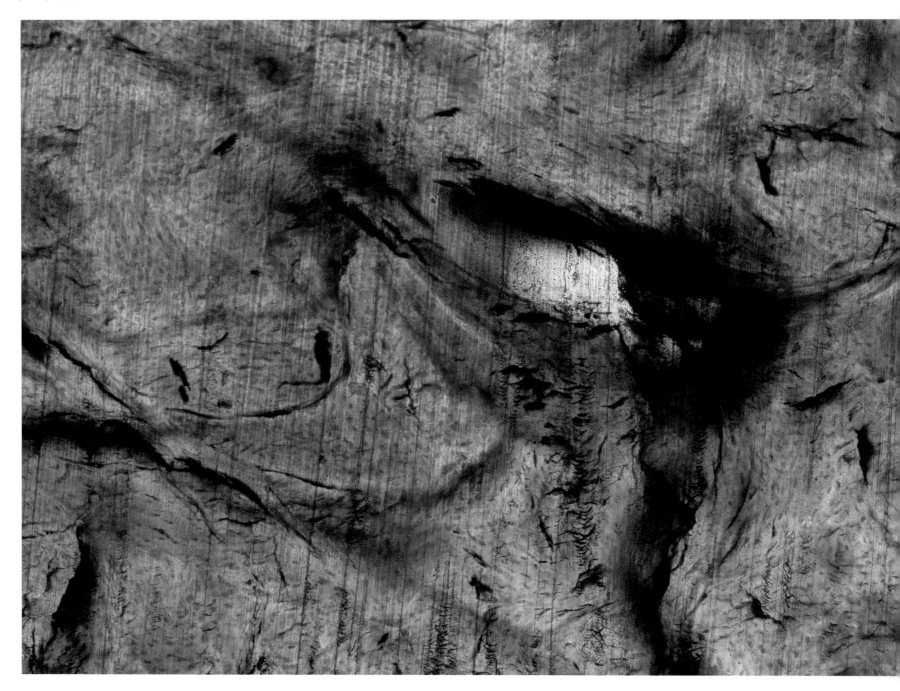

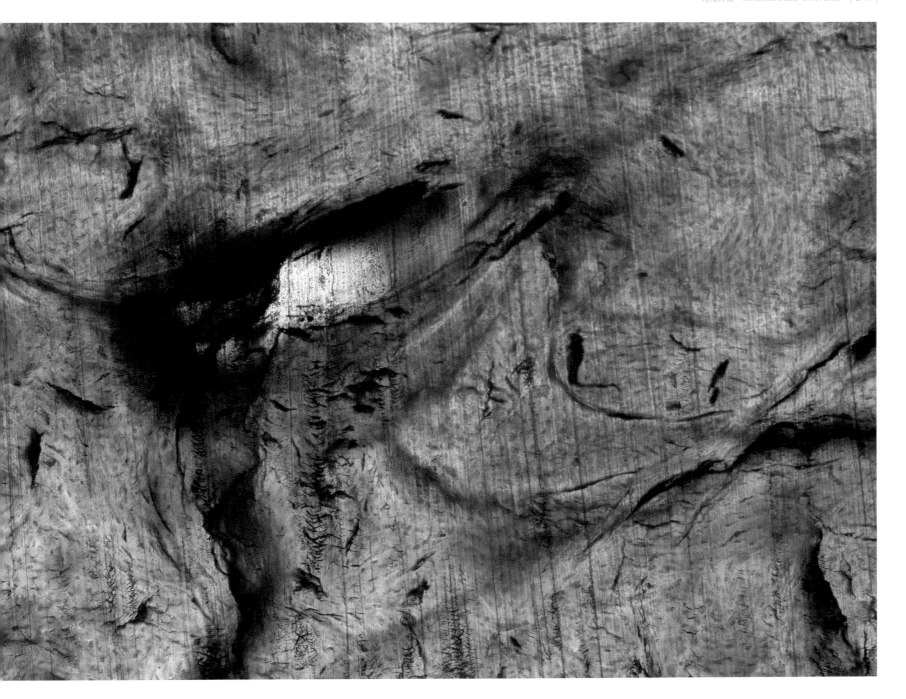

狮子王

未脱钙骨组织磨片的局部镜像，×200，明视野，2019

Lion King

Mirror image of part of cortical bone, Grounding tissue section, ×200, Light field, 2019

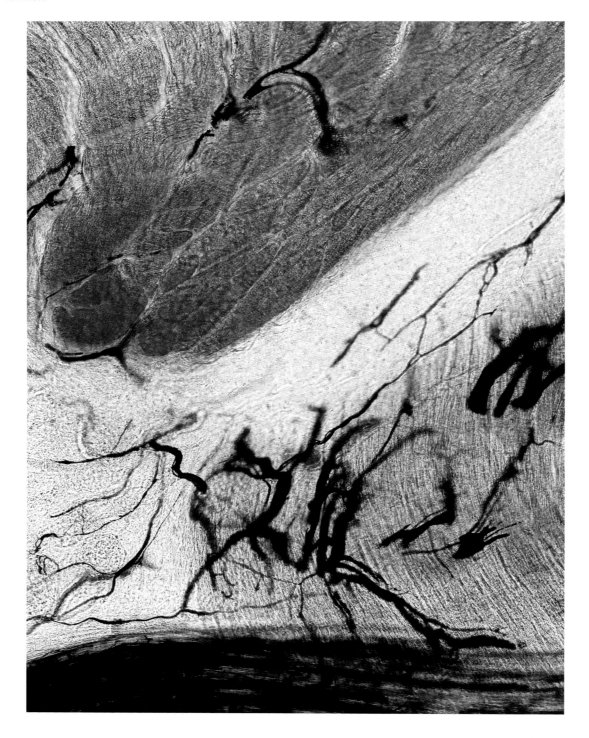

梦舞

灌墨血管组织切片，×40，明视野，2019

Dream Dance

Ink-irrigated blood vessels and muscles, Tissue section, ×40, Light field, 2019

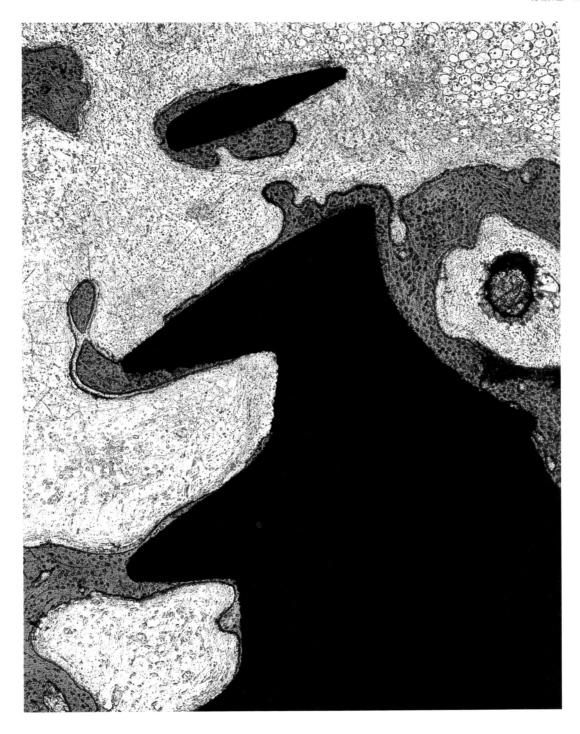

红衣裳

未脱钙骨组织和种植体磨片，×100，明视野 + 偏振光，2019

Red Clothes

Intersurface of implant and the bone, Hard tissue section of the jaw, ×100, Light field + polarized light, 2019

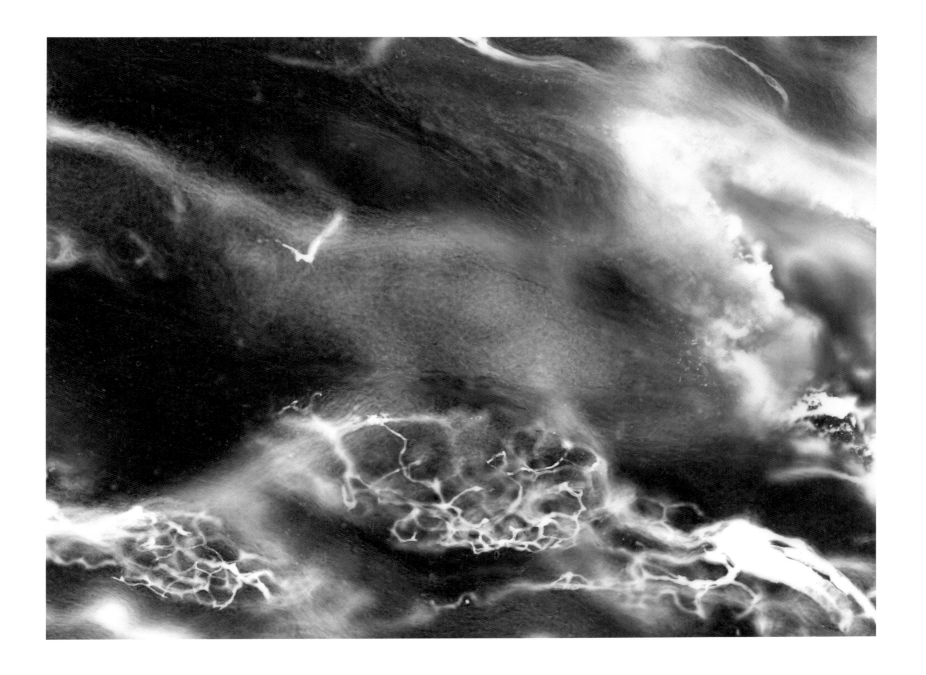

海的精灵

灌墨血管组织切片，×40，偏振光的负像，2014

Elf of the Sea

Ink-irrigated blood vessels, Tissue section, ×40, Negative image of polarized light, 2014

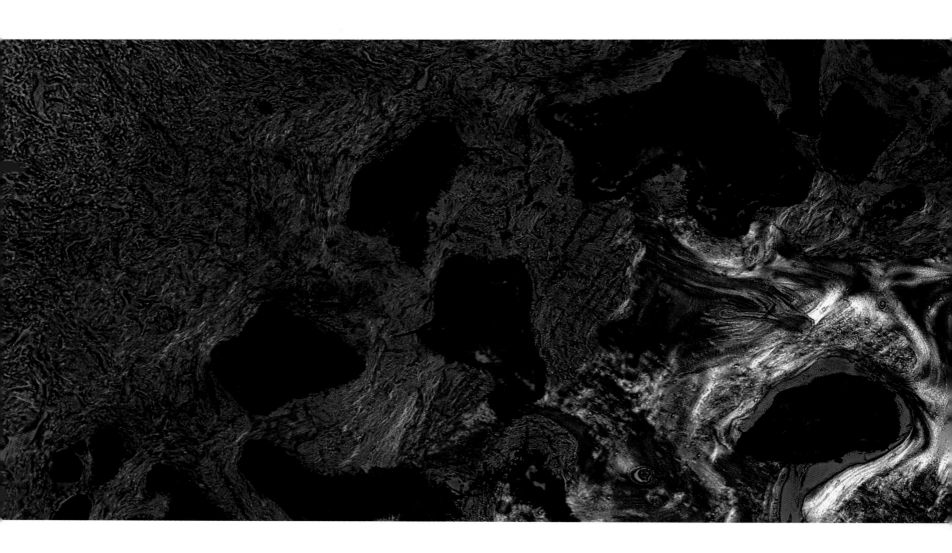

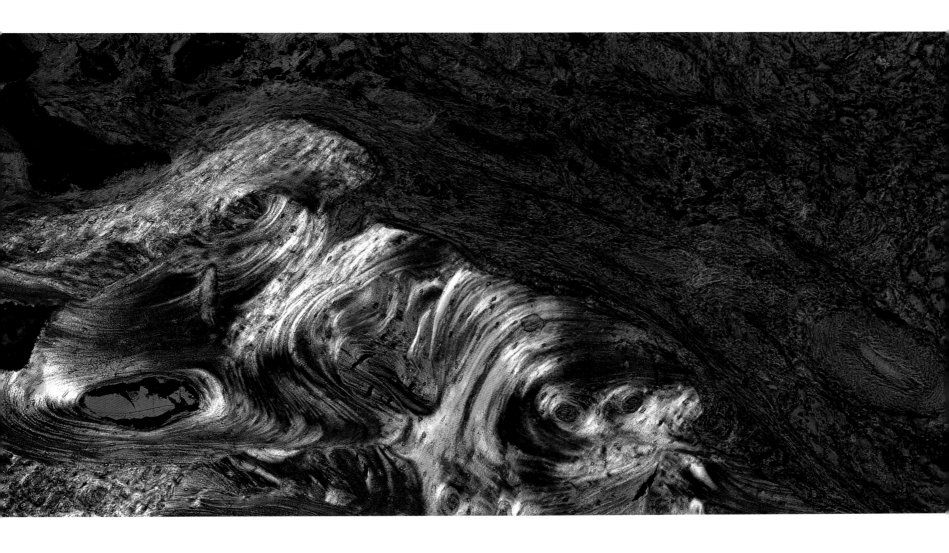

山舞银蛇
未脱钙骨及周围组织磨片，×100，偏振光，2019

Silver Snake Like Dancing Mountain
Bone and surrounding soft tissues, Grounding tissue section, ×100, Polarized light, 2019

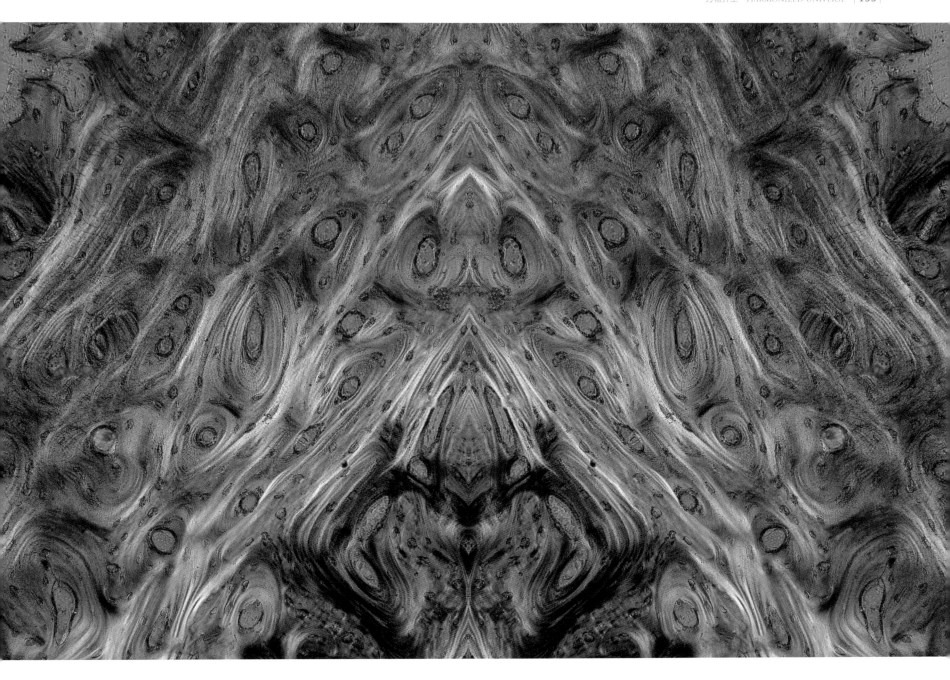

凤凰涅槃
未脱钙骨组织磨片的局部镜像，×200，偏振光，2019

Phoenix Nirvana
Mirror image of part of bone tissue, Grounding tissue section, ×200, Polarized light, 2019

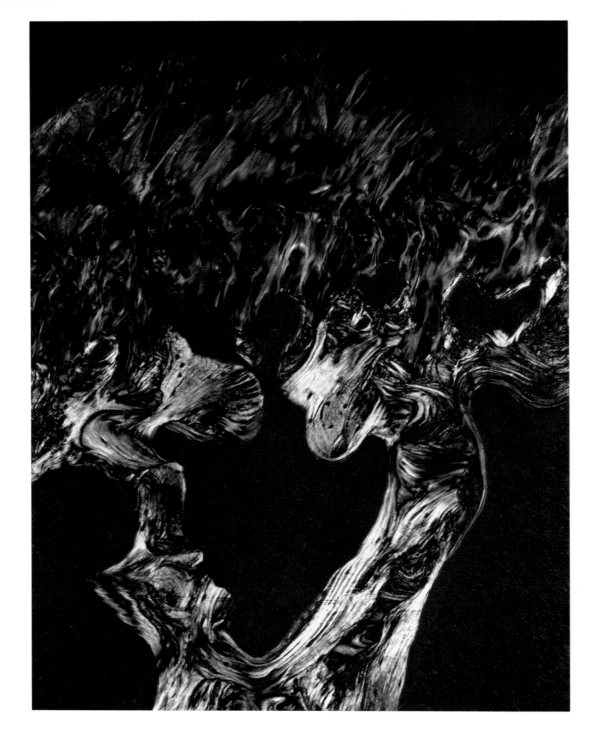

相守

脱钙髁突骨软骨组织切片，×100，偏振光，2019

Stay Together

Bone and cartilage tissues in the joint, Grounding tissue section, ×100, Polarized light, 2019

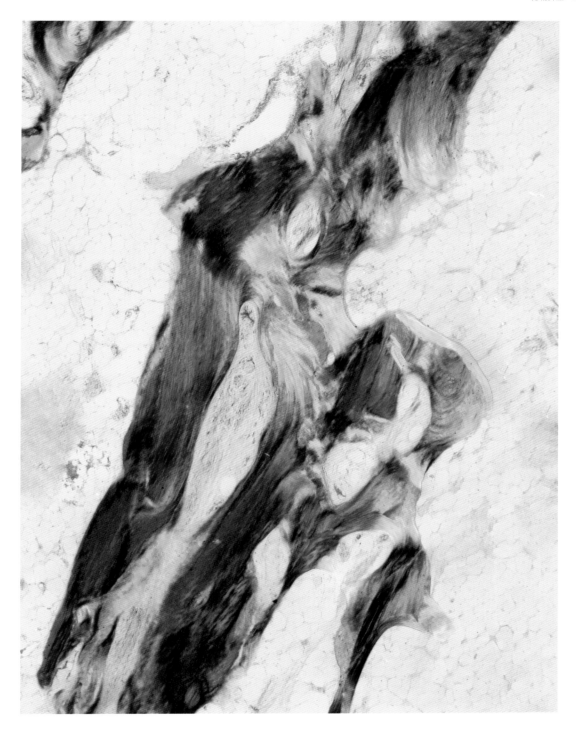

舞
脱钙骨组织切片，×100，明视野＋偏振光，2013

Dancing
Trabecular bone, Tissue section, ×100, Light field + polarized light, 2013

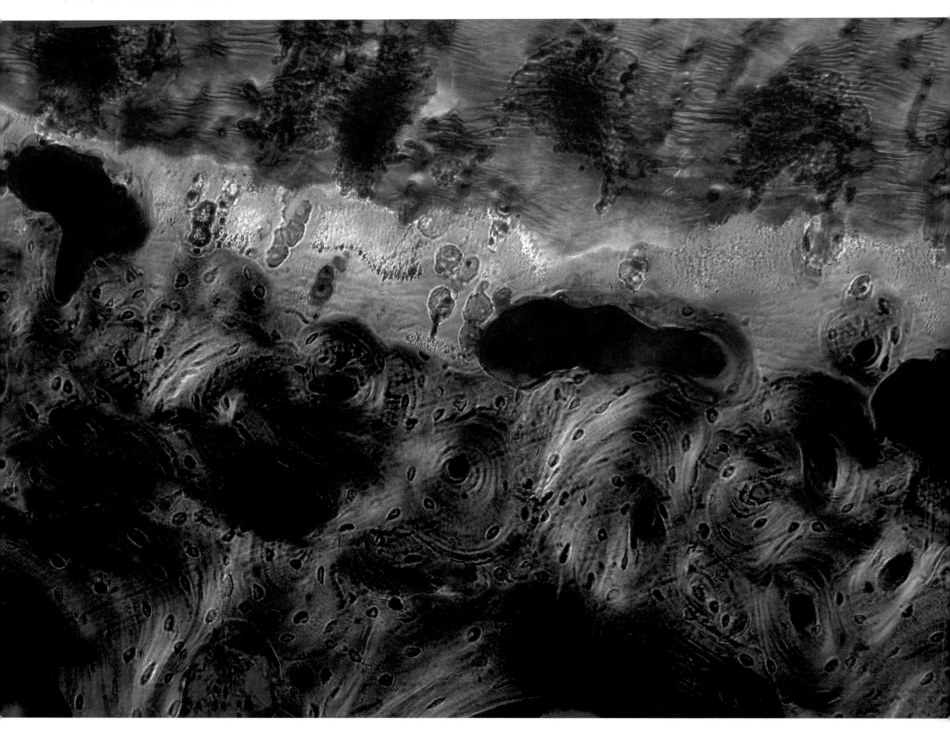

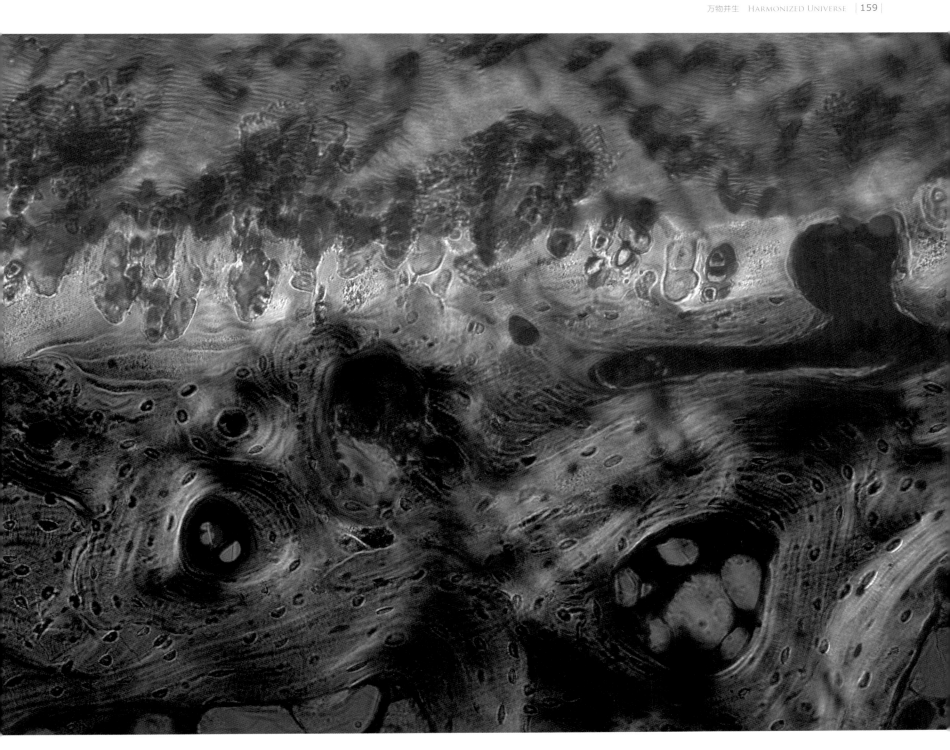

一半是海水

未脱钙骨组织磨片与树胶交界处，×100，明视野 + 偏振光，2019

Half is Sea Water

Bone tissue and the sealing gel, Grounding tissue section, ×100, Light field + polarized light, 2019

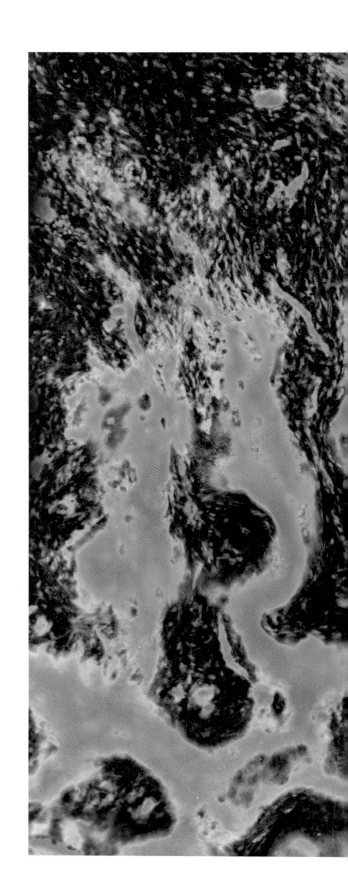

欢乐颂
脱钙骨组织切片的局部镜像，×40，明视野 + 偏振光，2014

Song of Joy
Mirror image of part of bone tissue section, ×40, Light field+polarized light, 2014

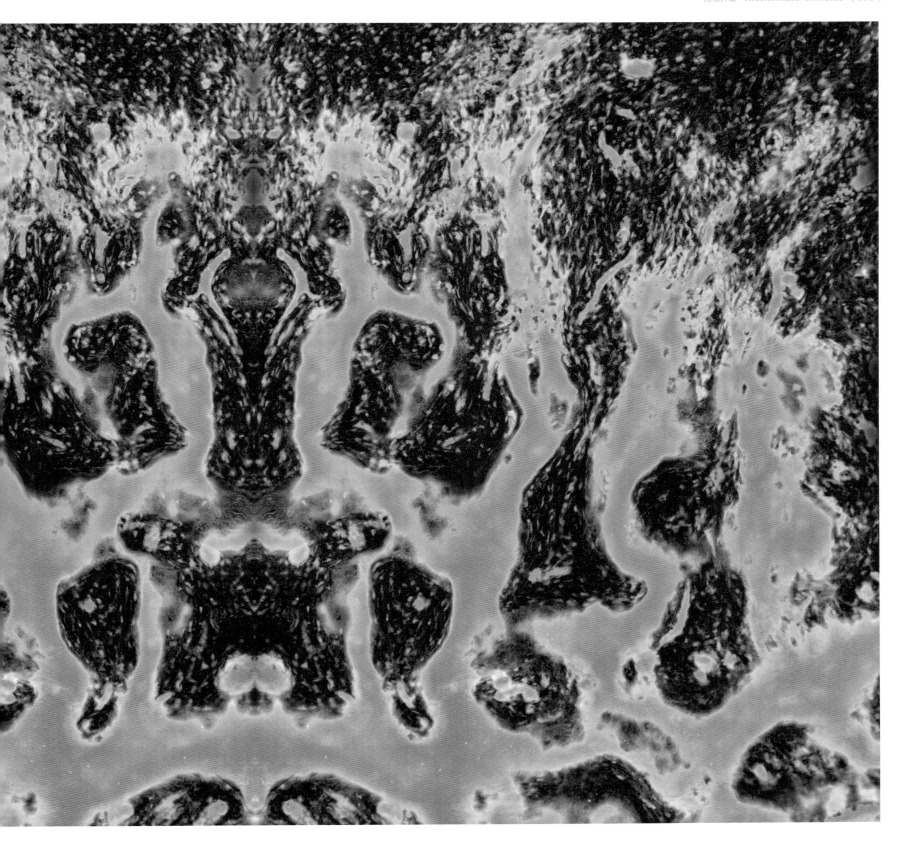

显微镜下的美丽相遇

《北医人》记者徐璐对李铁军教授的专题访谈

BEAUTIFUL ENCOUNTER UNDER THE MICROSCOPE

Special interview with Professor Li Tiejun by Xu Lu, a reporter from Periodical - *The Beiyiren*

2013 年 11 月，一场独特的展览在北医校园揭幕，这是口腔病理学专家李铁军教授的显微摄影作品展《生命如诗》。血管、肌肉组织、骨组织……这些在医学人眼中极其平常的事物，在李铁军的显微镜头下被重新发现，展现出其既熟悉又陌生，既真实又魔幻的艺术魅力。

医学部常务副主任柯杨在揭幕仪式上说："通过这些作品，让我们静心欣赏大自然的鬼斧神工及美感，感慨自然的创造力。通过对生命的感悟，提升医学人格。"医学人文研究院王一方教授说："李铁军教授以新的方式展示了病理学，通过有界与无界、有形与无形、有象与无象的结合，诠释了'医学不仅仅是技术，也是艺术的生存方向'的理念。"

In November 2013, a unique exhibition was unveiled on the campus of Peking University Health Science Center. This is the photomicrograph exhibition "Life in Poetry" by Professor Li Tiejun, an oral pathologist. Blood vessels, muscles, bone tissues... these things that are extremely common in the eyes of medical doctors and students have been rediscovered under Li Tiejun's microscope, showing their familiar and unfamiliar artistic charms that are both real and magical.

Ke Yang, executive deputy director of the Health Science Center, said at the opening ceremony, "Through these works, we can calmly appreciate the magical work and beauty of nature, as well as the creativity of nature. Through the perception of life, we can enhance our medical identity and professionalism." Professor Wang Yifang, from the Research Institute of Medical Humanities, said "Professor Li demonstrated pathology in a brand new way. Through the combination of boundary and crossover, tangible and intangible, concrete and abstract, he tried to explain the notion that medicine is not only about technology, but also about humanity and the art of survival."

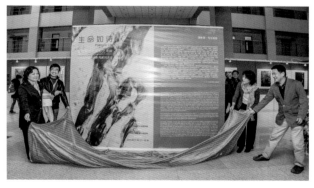

2013 年 11 月，北京大学医学部医学人文周"生命如诗"艺术展开幕式

In November 2013, Medical Humanities Week organized by Peking University Health Science Center, "Life in Poetry" art exhibition opening ceremony

世界上最失落的两个职业是牙医和摄影师：牙医想当医生，摄影师想成为画家。

—— 西班牙画家，巴勃罗·毕加索

The two most lost professions in the world are dentists and photographers: a dentist wants to become a doctor, and photographers want to be painters.

—— Spanish painter, Pablo Picasso

毕加索的这句话让李铁军很感兴趣，这句话刚好涵盖了他所从事的两个领域。"读到这句话时，我想到的是再伟大的大师也有他的时代局限性。现在的口腔医学早已不是过去的'镶牙匠'，现在的摄影也早被确立为独立的艺术门类。"

"口腔病理学家"和"摄影师"，当这两个词并列放在一起时，有一种"大学里走错课堂"的感觉。而在李铁军身上，这一切发生得又是那么顺其自然。

This words of Picasso made Li Tiejun very interested, and it happened to cover the two fields he was engaged in. "When I read this sentence, what I thought was that no matter how great a master is, he has the limitations of his time. Today's stomatology is no longer the 'dentist' of the past, and today's photography has long been established as an independent art category."

"Oral pathologist" and "photographer", when these two labels are placed side by side, you may feel like entering a "wrong class" in an university. However, when it does happen in Li Tiejun, all this happened so naturally.

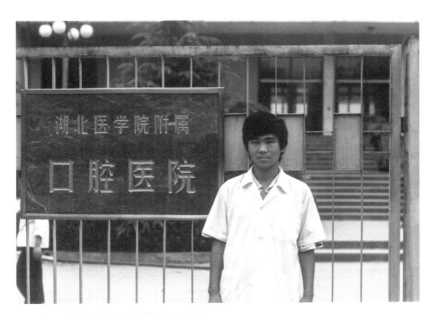

1982 年，湖北医学院口腔系本科实习生

In 1982, undergraduate intern in Faculty of Stomatology, Hubei Medical College

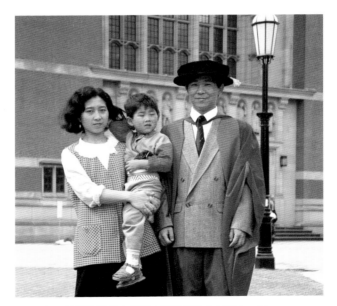

1995 年，英国伯明翰大学博士毕业典礼上与家人一起

In 1995, with family members at the PhD graduation ceremony at the University of Birmingham, UK

从"艺术青年"到"医学青年"

李铁军从事口腔病理学专业三十年，在颌骨牙源性肿瘤临床与基础研究领域颇有成就。但有趣的是，无论是学医、学口腔、学病理都不是李铁军当时的第一选择。

儿时，李铁军从未想过，自己将来要去当一名医生。尽管他从小在部队医院长大，尽管他的父母都是医务工作者，李铁军却对绘画感兴趣，他常常背着画板，和小伙伴们一起去学画。

高考恢复后，父母建议他"放下画笔，复习考试"。李铁军听从父母的意见，考入湖北医学院口腔系（现武汉大学口腔医学院）。"当时报考的是医疗系，后来分到了口腔系。"

李铁军的人生轨迹开始了一个巨大的转折，手中的画笔变成解剖刀，画板上的斑斓色彩变成厚厚教科书里的医学术语。

从"艺术青年"转变到"医学青年"，李铁军倒是没有太大的不适应。"我个人觉得医科和文科是很接近的。虽然把它归属于理科，但更多的时候，我们是在和文字打交道，比如说读书、与患者交流、写论文等。"

大学期间，李铁军成绩优异，他最喜欢口腔修复学，本想着将来当一名镶牙医生。"可能因为修复、镶牙也跟美学相关吧。"但读研时，李铁军考取了口腔病理学研究生。"当时只允许应届毕业生考基础学科的研究生，因为我们没有临床经验。"

之后，李铁军去英国读博，到日本做博士后，回国后在北大口腔医院成为一名病理科医生，一路走下来，李铁军在口腔病理学领域越钻越深。

From "artistic youth" to "medical doctor"

Li Tiejun has been engaged in oral pathology for 30 years and has made considerable achievements in the field of clinical and basic research on odontogenic tumors of the jaws. But what is interesting is that neither studying medicine, stomatology, or pathology was Li Tiejun's first choice at the time.

When he was a child, Li Tiejun never thought that he would become a doctor in the future. Although he grew up in a military hospital and his parents were both medical workers, Li Tiejun was interested in painting. He often carried a drawing board and went to learn painting with his friends.

After the national university entrance examination resumed in the late 1970's, his parents suggested that he should put down the paintbrush and start to prepare for the exam. Li Tiejun listened to his parents' opinions and was admitted to the School of Stomatology of Hubei Medical College (now known as Wuhan University School of Stomatology). "At that time, I applied for the clinical medicine, but I was then assigned to the dental school."

Li Tiejun's life track has appeared a huge turning point. The paintbrush in his hand has become a scalpel, and the colorful colors on the drawing board have become medical terms in thick textbooks.

Li Tiejun didn't feel too uncomfortable to change from "art youth" to "medical student". "I personally think that medicine and liberal arts are in fact very close in nature. Although medicine belongs to the category of science, more often we are dealing with words, such as reading, communicating with patients, and writing papers."

During college, Li had excellent grades. Among all the specialties in stomatology, he liked prosthodontics the most, and he wanted to be a prosthodontist in the future. "Maybe because dental restoration is more related to aesthetics." But when he was in graduate school, Li Tiejun was admitted to the postgraduate of oral pathology. "At that time, the recent graduates were only allowed to take the examination for graduate students in basic disciplines because we had no clinical experience."

Later, Li Tiejun went to the UK to study for a Ph.D., and then went to Japan as a postdoctoral fellow. After returning to China, he became a pathologist at the Peking University School of Stomatology. All the way, Li Tiejun got deeper and deeper in the field of oral pathology.

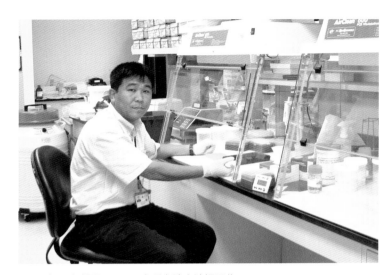

2004 年，在美国 UTMB 病理实验室访问工作

Visiting scholar in pathology laboratory at UTMB, USA, in 2004

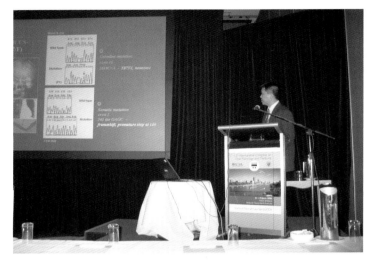

2006 年，在第 13 届国际口腔病理学年会上发言（布里斯班，澳大利亚）

In 2006, speaking at the 13th annual conference of International Association of Oral Pathology (Brisbane, Australia)

"口腔临床分支很广，不同的临床专业所用的理论、术语差异很大，而口腔病理恰恰是一个桥梁学科，能把临床各专业及基础学科相链接。因此口腔病理在口腔医学中是很重要的，也很有趣。"

正是因为这样的一种桥梁学科地位，作为病理科医生的李铁军不满足于日常的诊断工作，还用较多的时间从事科研工作。

"我的性格是'从一而终'型的，虽然不是因为热爱而去学病理，但一旦进入了，找到兴趣了，就想'一条路走到底'。我喜欢病理，做合格的病理大夫一直是我的追求。"

李铁军的主要研究方向是颌骨牙源性病损的生长特点和临床行为，他于 2006 年获得国家杰出青年科学基金，2010 年他应口腔医学领域的顶级杂志《Journal of Dental Research》主编的邀请，撰写有关牙源性角化囊肿的研究综述，足以见其在此领域的学术地位。

"Oral clinical branches are numerous, and the theories and terminology used by different clinical specialties are very different. Oral pathology is just a bridge discipline that can link clinical specialties and basic disciplines. Therefore, oral pathology is very important in stomatology, and it's also very interesting."

It is because of such a feature as a bridge discipline that Li Tiejun, as a pathologist, is not satisfied with daily diagnostic work and spends more time engaged in scientific research.

"My personality is of the 'one to the end' type. Although I didn't go to study pathology because of my first choice, once I entered the specialty and found interest, I wanted to go all the way to the end. I like pathology and to become a qualified pathologist has always been my pursuit."

Li Tiejun's main research interest is the growth and behavior of odontogenic lesions of the jaws. He was awarded the National Science Fund for Outstanding Young Scholars in 2006. In 2010, he was invited by the editor-in-chief of Journal of Dental Research, the top journal in the field of dentistry, to write a review on recent research development in odontogenic keratocyst. All these maybe a reflection of his academic status in his professional field.

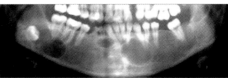

CRITICAL REVIEWS IN ORAL BIOLOGY & MEDICINE

T.-J. Li

Department of Oral Pathology, Peking University School and Hospital of Stomatology, 22 South Zhongguancun Avenue, Haidian District, Beijing 100081, PR China; litiejun22@vip.sina.com

J Dent Res 90(2):133-142, 2011

The Odontogenic Keratocyst: A Cyst, or a Cystic Neoplasm?

ABSTRACT

The odontogenic keratocyst (OKC, currently designated by the World Health Organization as a keratocystic odontogenic tumor) is a locally aggressive, cystic jaw lesion with a putative high growth potential and a propensity for recurrence. Although it is generally agreed that some features of OKCs are those of a neoplasia, notably the relatively high proliferative rate of epithelial cells, controversies over the behavior and management of OKCs still exist. This article is intended to review this intriguing entity and to summarize the findings of recent studies related to the nature of OKCs and their clinical and therapeutic implications. Recent advances in genetic and molecular research, i.e., PTCH1 mutations and involvement of the Hedgehog signaling pathway, have led to increased knowledge of OKC pathogenesis which hints at potential new treatment options, although the question of whether the OKC is a cyst or a cystic neoplasm is yet to be answered with certainty. Since some advocate a more conservative treatment for OKCs, notably marsupialization and decompression, future treatment strategies may focus on molecular approaches and eventually reduce or eliminate the need for aggressive surgeries.

INTRODUCTION

The term 'odontogenic keratocyst' (OKC) was first introduced by Philipsen over 50 years ago to describe a group of odontogenic cysts which showed a characteristic histological appearance (Philipsen, 1956). As compared with other types of odontogenic cysts, OKCs appear to have an intrinsically higher growth potential (Main, 1970; Browne, 1971; Li et al., 1993, 1994a,b). A propensity to recur following surgical treatment, a relationship to the so-called 'Gorlin syndrome' (also known as nevoid basal cell carcinoma syndrome), and the potential risk of neoplastic change place OKCs in a unique position within the spectrum of odontogenic lesions. It has long been suggested that OKCs should be regarded as benign neoplasms (Ahlfors et al., 1984; Shear, 2002a,b). While the first 2 WHO classifications of odontogenic lesions (Pindborg et al., 1971; Kramer et al., 1992) put OKCs into the category of developmental odontogenic cysts, the most recent edition designates the OKC as a keratocystic odontogenic tumor (Barnes et al., 2005), implying that the lesion is a benign neoplasm. This new classification and terminology have aroused heated debates over the nature of OKCs, particularly among oral and maxillofacial surgeons and pathologists. Although considerable insight into the biological profile of the OKC has been accumulated in recent years (Gomes et al., 2009a; Mendes et al., 2010), controversies over its behavior and management still exist. The question of whether the OKC is a cyst or a

发表于《牙科研究杂志》的综述

Invited review published in *Journal of Dental Research*

8-9B. Odontogenic keratocyst

Speight P.
Devilliers P.
Li T.-J.
Odell E.W.
Wright J.M.

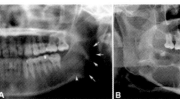

Definition
Odontogenic keratocyst (OKC) is an odontogenic cyst characterized by a thin, regular lining of parakeratinized stratified squamous epithelium with palisading hyperchromatic basal cells.

Synonym
Keratocystic odontogenic tumour

Epidemiology
OKCs account for 10–20% of odontogenic cysts and are the third most common cyst of the jaws {1145,1149}. They occur over a wide patient age range, with a peak incidence in the second to third decades of life and a second, smaller peak among patients aged 50–70 years {1149}. Most studies find a slight male predilection {2153}. As many as 5% of all OKCs occur as part of naevoid basal cell carcinoma syndrome (Gorlin syndrome) {1419}; these cases tend to be multiple and to occur in younger patients {2638}.

Fig. 3458 Odontogenic keratocyst. A patient with naevoid basal cell carcinoma syndrome with multiple odontogenic keratocysts in the mandible and maxilla.

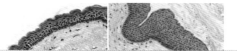

Fig. 3456, 3457 Odontogenic keratocyst. **A** A unilocular radiolucency at the angle of the mandible extending to the posterior aspect of the ramus (arrows). **B** An extensive multilocular lesion from the midline, filling the body of the mandible and extending into the ramus; the lesions are well demarcated and mostly corticated.

参编《WHO 头颈肿瘤分类》

Contributor to *WHO Classification of Head and Neck Tumours*

"可能我比较执着吧，不嫌这个领域冷，不嫌小，始终做下去，时间长了就成了专家了。"对于成绩，李铁军这样说。

如今已是口腔病理专家的李铁军，更在显微摄影的艺术领域走出了一片自己的天地。

回顾以往，李铁军这样总结："现在来看，是各种机遇、机缘促成了我今天的职业道路；而站在我当时的视角，更多地可能是无奈。但生活是圆的，你无意的选择和你内心的追求，有的时候会契合。"

"Maybe I am quite persistent. I don't think this field is too small or unpopular. I just keep doing it. After a long time, I will become an expert." Li Tiejun commented on his own achievements.

Li Tiejun, now an expert in oral pathology, has made his own way to pioneer the artistic presentation of microphotography.

Looking back on the past, Li Tiejun said "Looking at it now, various opportunities, mostly unexpected, have contributed to my career path today; and at the time from my perspective, it may be not at all satisfying. But life is round. The choice that you have no intention to make and the pursuit within your own heart sometimes fit each other well."

科学家是用所有人都熟悉的语言，讲述从没有人知道的知识；而诗人用从没有人用过的语言，表达人人都会有的感情。

—— 英国理论物理学家，保罗·狄拉克

Scientists use language familiar to everyone to tell knowledge that no one has ever known; while poets use language that no one has ever used to express feelings that everyone has.

—— British theoretical physicist, Paul Dirac

跨界的探索

"艺术是寻美，科学是求真。"李铁军将"求真"所用的显微镜作为照相机的镜头去"寻美"，这无疑是一次"跨界"探索。

第一次看显微镜时，李铁军就被眼前这个奇妙的微观世界打动了。"肉眼看到的东西常常是司空见惯的，突然有这样的科学仪器辅助你，见到平时未曾见过的，这带给我一种艺术般的视觉感受。"

此时，显微镜带给李铁军的艺术遐想只是零星的、偶然的、一过性的。"最初，显微摄影是需要胶片的，很贵，所以几乎所有的显微照片都是做科研和讲课用的。"李铁军是一名整天与显微镜打交道的医学人。数十年来，他的日常工作就是通过显微镜观察组织、细胞的形态特点和变化，辅助对疾病的诊断。

这项工作重要且责任重大，"常常要经历'生'与'死'的判断和考量"。李铁军说："在日积月累地与不同生命个体接触、交流过程中，病理医师可能会有更多的哲学思考，因为不仅要了解患者的临床表现，还要去探究许多肉眼看不到的变化。"

业余时间里，李铁军是一名"摄影发烧友"。在难得的节假日里，他会起早贪黑捕捉美景。"学医之后，没有太多的时间和机会再去画画。近年来，随着数码相机的普及，摄影变得方便、快捷，成为人人可及的艺术体验。对于我来说，镜头越来越像画笔、快门越来越像灵感一现。"

Cross-border exploration

"Art is seeking beauty, science is seeking truth." Li Tiejun uses the microscope used in "seeking truth" as the lens of a camera to "see beauty". This is undoubtedly a "cross-border" exploration.

When he first looked at the microscope, Li Tiejun was moved by the wonderful microscopic world in front of him. "It is common to see things with the naked eye. Suddenly there is such a scientific instrument to assist you. Seeing things you have never seen before gives me an artistic visual experience."

At that time, the artistic reverie that the microscope brought to Li Tiejun was only sporadic, accidental, and transient. "In the beginning, photomicrography needed films, which was very expensive, so almost all photomicrographs were used for scientific research and lectures." Li Tiejun is a doctor who deals with microscopes all day. For decades, his daily work has been to observe the morphological characteristics and changes of tissues and cells through a microscope to assist in the diagnosis of diseases.

This work is important and full of responsibility. "It often has to experience the judgment and consideration of life and death." Li said, "In the process of accumulating contact and communicating with different living individuals, pathologists may have more philosophical thinking, because they not only must understand the clinical manifestations of patients, but also have to explore many invisible changes to the naked eye."

In his spare time, Li Tiejun is a "photographer amateur". On holidays, he would get up early in the morning or stay late till dusk to capture the natural beauty. "After studying medicine, there is not much time and opportunity to

"摄影作品捕捉到的瞬间，不是简单的 copy 自然景观，而是经过你内心思考和凝练后，呈现给观者的影像。即所谓，你拍摄的风景是你内心的风景。"李铁军在摄影时，努力追求的是一种别人似见未见的"陌生感"。

带着这种体会，李铁军对显微镜下的影像进行了重新思考，显微影像不正有一种与生俱来的"陌生感"吗？"摄影是截取生活的片段，而病理切片的过程实际也是截取组织的过程，两者都是取舍的艺术。"

paint. In recent years, with the popularization of digital cameras, photography has become convenient and fast, and it has become an artistic experience accessible to everyone. For me, the camera lens is becoming more and more like a brush, and the shutter is more like a flash of inspiration."

"The moment captured by the photographic work is not a simple copy of the natural landscape, but the image presented to the audience through your inner thinking and composing. That is to say, the scenery you shoot is the scenery in your heart." When taking photos, Li strives for a sense of "strangeness" that others seem to have never seen.

With this kind of experience, Li Tiejun rethinks the image under the microscope. Doesn't the microscope image have an inherent sense of "strangeness"? "Photography is to intercept fragments of life, and the process of pathological sectioning is actually the process of intercepting tissues. Both are the art of focusing and capture."

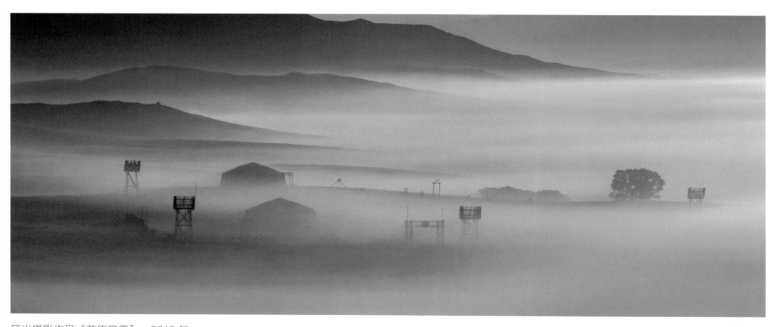

风光摄影作品"草原晨雾"，2013 年

Landscape photography "Morning Mist in the Prairie", 2013

也许是数十年来从医和科研的经历，也许是儿时的美术功底练就的对影像的敏感，李铁军对显微镜下的形态、色彩和光影有了更多的思考和联想。"在这些看似平常的组织切片中，我常常可以捕捉到生物体的变幻莫测和活灵活现，常常能产生很多奇思妙想。比如说，在低倍镜下浏览组织切片时，会有一种从飞机上航拍大地的错觉；在明视野下观察各类染色切片时，会联想起缤纷的四季；在暗视野下捕捉荧光的细胞或组织定位时，会惊叹镜下的光影变幻无异于夜色的灵透与神秘……"

Perhaps it was his experience in medicine and scientific research for decades, or his sensitivity to images acquired through his childhood art experiences, Li Tiejun has more thoughts and imaginations about the shape, color, light and shadow of the human tissues under the microscope. "In these seemingly ordinary tissue sections, I can often capture the unpredictable and vivid life of cells and tissues, and can often produce some whimsical ideas. For example, when browsing tissue slides under a low power microscope, there will be a kind of illusion that we overlook the earth from an airplane; when observing various kinds of stained sections in bright field, you will think of the colorful four seasons; when you capture fluorescence in cells or tissues in dark field, you will be amazed that the light and shadow changes under the microscope are no different from the mysterious and beautiful night..."

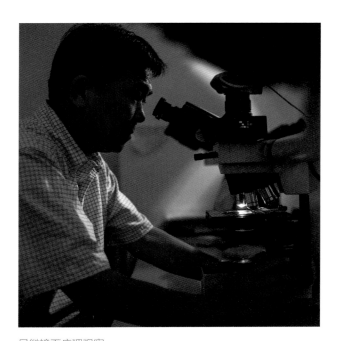

显微镜下病理观察

Pathological observation under microscope

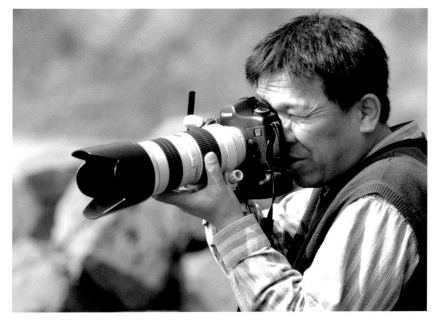

外出摄影采风

Go outing and take pictures

通过特殊染色、棱镜变化、构图，李铁军将组织内的"美景"提炼出来。这种"美景"即便在医学人士眼中，也不再是司空见惯的组织、结构，而有了一种"非医学"的陌生感；而普通人由于没有医学背景，观看显微影像便有与大自然景观似曾相识的感觉。李铁军把这种跨界带来的"陌生与熟悉"称之为"否定之否定"的视觉思维过程。

Through special staining, prism changes, and composition, Li Tiejun extracts the "beauty" in the tissues or organs. Even in the eyes of medical professionals, this "beauty" is no longer a common tissue structure, but has a sense of "non-medical" strangeness; while ordinary people have no medical background, watching microscopic images is more like enjoying the natural landscape that one feels more familiar. Li Tiejun calls the "strangeness and familiarity" brought about by this cross-border exploration as the visual thinking process of "negation of negation".

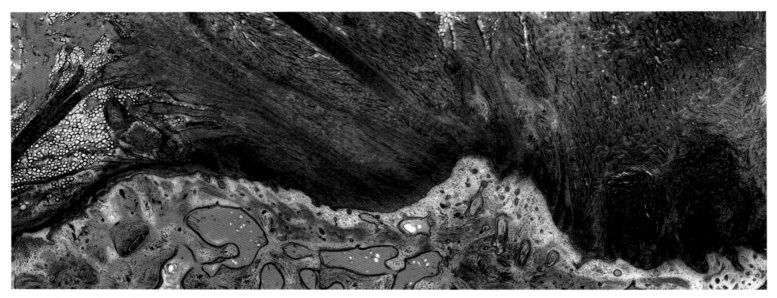

显微摄影作品"秋色漫山"，骨及肌肉组织磨片，2019 年

Photomicrograph "Autumn in the Mountains", bone and muscle tissue grounding section, 2019

李铁军在显微摄影方面的探索受到了各方的好评，摄影圈的专业老师们更是对此感叹神奇，鼓励他探索其中奥秘。"这是我的意外惊喜和收获，也开始认真研究显微摄影的技术沿革和独特魅力，系统梳理我多年来拍摄收集的显微影像，审视这些生命微像所蕴含的无限生机和精神力量。"

Li Tiejun's exploration in photomicrography has been well received by many, and even the professional photographers sighed for the magic and encouraged him to explore this field further. "This is my unexpected surprise, so I have begun to seriously study the technological evolution and unique charm of photomicrography, systematically sort out the microscopic images I have taken and collected over the years, and look into the infinite vitality and spiritual power hidden in these micro-images of life. "

2014 年初，李铁军的显微摄影集——《生命之美》出版，书中收录他 97 幅显微摄影作品，分"混沌初开""万物生长""静水流深""生生不息""天人合一"五个主题，从生命物质本源的微细结构，展示生命之魅力。

At the beginning of 2014, Li Tiejun's photomicrograph collection album — *The Beauty of Life* was published. The book collected 97 photomicrographs of him and displayed with five themes including "Chaotic Genesis" "All Things Grow" "Still Water Flows Deep" "Flourish Life" and "Harmony between Human and Nature". The book shows the charm of life from the fine structures constituting the origin of life itself.

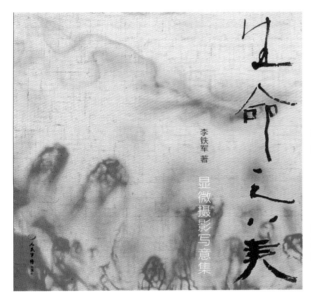

《生命之美》封面，2014 年

The cover of *The Beauty of Life*, 2014

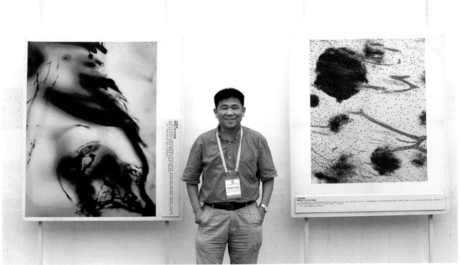

2013 年，参加第五届全国科技摄影展

In 2013, participation in the 5th national science and technology photography exhibition

在书的后记中，李铁军写道："艺术的写意，似乎背离了科学求真务实的目的，这也许是一种探索吧，一种实验，一种希望让科学与艺术相融合的尝试。我分不清楚这其中的是与非，但我很喜欢这种跨界的相遇过程。"

In the book's postscript, Li Tiejun wrote: "The freehand brushwork of art seems to deviate from the purpose of seeking truth and being pragmatic in science. This may be an exploration, an experiment, an attempt to integrate science and art. I admit that I am not sure about the right and wrong of this, but I really enjoy the process of this kind of cross-border encounter."

医学是不确定的科学与可能性的艺术。

——加拿大医学家、教育家，威廉·奥斯勒

Medicine is the art of uncertain science and possibility.

—— Canadian medical scientist and educator, William Osler

科学与艺术在山顶相遇

李铁军不是传统意义上的工作狂，工作之外他兴趣很多。但他做事投入，讲效率，热爱起来，不知疲倦。身兼医院党务、行政职务，工作日中的李铁军往往事务缠身、忙碌异常，周末成了他做科研、拍片子的最好时间。在显微镜前，他常常一坐就是一整天。

"我曾经觉得自己这样执着地在显微影像中'寻美'，会不会是'节外生枝'，偏离了职业轨道。"李铁军坦言他曾经的犹豫和纠结，但北京大学医学人文研究院王一方教授的评论让他得以释怀。

"医学与艺术的对话，可以互相汲取生命的感悟、培育生命的灵感与技术的创造力，更高的境界是医生在艺术上登堂入室，径直闯入艺术的价值殿堂，去尝试艺术化生存的人生境界。艺术让医生对痛苦、死亡的理解和领悟更加深刻，不仅仅只是躯体的病变与恶化，而是对待生命的姿态，爱的秩序，价值的位序，引领医者去感知'厚道'，逼近崇高，抵达神圣。"在李铁军摄影展的前言中，王一方如此评论。

王一方教授直言，中国的医学教育正需要李铁军这样的老师。

现代医学的发展，越来越多地启示我们，医生要跳出"技术中心论"的藩篱，回归"以人为本"的本质。在北大医学部的教学改革中，对医学人文教育的重视程度也日益提升。

Science and art meet at the top of the mountain

Li Tiejun is not a workaholic in the traditional sense, he has a lot of interests outside of work. But he is committed to work, efficiently, whole-heartedly and tirelessly. As an administrative as well as a professional faculty in a hospital, Li Tiejun is often troubled and busy during workdays. Weekends have become his best time for scientific research and filming. In front of the microscope, he often sits all day.

"I once felt that I was so persistent in 'seeking beauty' in microscopic images. Could it be 'extraordinary branches' and deviated from the professional track." Li Tiejun admitted his hesitation and entanglement, but professor Wang Yifang, from the Research Institute of Medical Humanities, Peking University, commented on his cross-border activity which relieved him.

"The dialogue between medicine and art can enhance each other's perceptions of life, cultivate inspiration and technical creativity. The higher realm is that doctors go straight into the palace of art's value, and try to experience an artistic life. Art allows doctors to understand and comprehend pain and death more deeply. To face a patient as a doctor, it is not only about the disease and deterioration of the body, but also the attitude towards life, the value of love. It also leads the doctors to perceive higher moral standard of 'kindness' which is sublime and sacred."

Professor Wang Yifang commented in the preface of Li Tiejun's photo exhibition and said bluntly that Chinese medical education needs teachers like Li Tiejun.

The development of modern medicine has increasingly enlightened us that doctors should break out of the barriers of "technology-centric theory" and return to the essence of "people-oriented care". In the teaching reform of Peking University Health Science Center, the emphasis on medical humanities education is increasing.

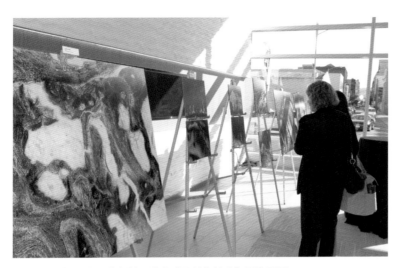

2016 年，美国太平洋大学牙学院"牙科的艺术"展览现场

"The Art of Dentistry" exhibition at the School of Dentistry, University of the Pacific, USA, 2016

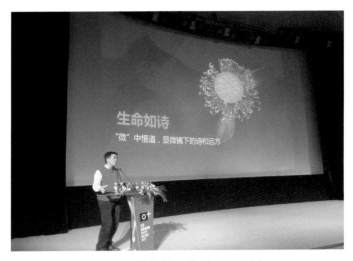

2017 年，北京国际摄影周"生命如诗"邀请展及讲座

In 2017, Beijing International Photography Week, "Life as poetry" invited exhibition and lecture

在大学读书期间，李铁军有两个"朋友圈"，一个是学医同学的"医学圈"，一个是学音乐、美术朋友的"艺术圈"。"当时我觉得他们学艺术的真好啊，心里难过时，就往琴房里一坐，弹出来的是自己的心情，我们就没有这样的表达方式。我们学医的烦了，只好去背几个单词、记几个术语，没有别的方法排遣。"

现在，李铁军每年都给在校的口腔医学生做有关显微影像美学趣味的讲座，很受欢迎。"人体内组织细胞的美和大自然中的美是一样的，个体的生老病死和大自然的沧桑变幻也是相互关联的。"他希望医学生通过人体组织内的微观世界去体会生命，体悟哲学中的"道法自然、天人合一"。

During his university student years, Li Tiejun had two "circles of friends", one was the "medical circle" of medical students, and the other was the "art circle" of music and painting art friends. "At that time, I admired the art students very much. When they felt sad, they sat in the piano room and played their own mood. But we medical students didn't have the luck to experience this way of expression. When we were bored, we had no other way but to read the textbooks and to memorize a few more words and terms."

Now, Li Tiejun gives lectures on the aesthetics of microscopic imaging to the students at school every year, which are very popular. "The beauty of the tissue cells in the human body is the same as the beauty of nature. The birth, aging, illness and death of individuals are also reflected in the vicissitudes of nature." He hopes that medical students can perceive life through observing the microcosm of human tissues and realize the philosophy of "Taoism" which believes that humans and nature are harmonized as one.

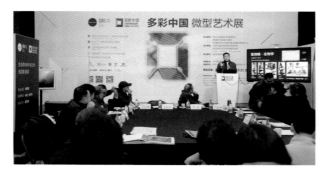

2018 年，在多彩中国微型艺术展"生命的科学与艺术"沙龙上发言

In 2018, speaking at the salon of "Science and Art of Life", Contemporary China – 10×12 art exhibition

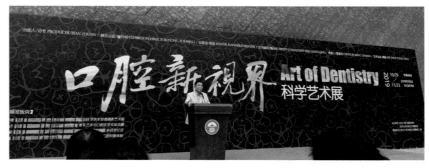

2019 年，在武汉大学万林艺术博物馆"口腔新视界"科学艺术展开幕式上发言

In 2019, speaking at the opening ceremony of the "New Oral Vision" science and art exhibition at Wanlin Art Museum of Wuhan University

　　"一名医师的成长过程，绝不仅仅是增长医术，在日积月累地与不同的生命个体的接触、交流过程中，一名医师同时应成长为患者的一位朋友，能够去尊重、安抚病人，让他对未来建立信心和希望，这是因为医师对生命有了更为全面和深刻的理解。"李铁军说。

　　学生们在课后的反馈中写到："原来单调、繁琐的医学生活中，也可以时有美的闪烁。"

　　李铁军对学生说："之所以认为科学与艺术互不往来、不相通，那是因为你站在一座山的两个山坡下，不管你的职业在哪个坡，都要努力攀登，等你到达山顶时，你会发现，心中那个对立面在山峰处与你是非常契合的。"

"The process of training a doctor is not just about to practice medical skills. Accumulating contact and communicating with different living individuals, a doctor should become a friend of the patient, and thus is able to respect and comfort them. This could enable the patient to build confidence and hope for the future. Therefore, the doctor is required to have a more comprehensive and profound understanding of life." Li Tiejun said.

His students wrote in their after-class feedback: "In the original monotonous and tedious medical life, there can also be flashes of beauty from time to time."

Li Tiejun said to the students: "The reason why you think that science and art are not interlinked or interrelated is because you are standing at the bottom of a mountain, which prevents you from seeing the other side. No matter which slope your career is on, you have to climb hard until you reach the top of the mountain and to see the opposite. At that time, you will find that the opposite slope hidden in your heart fits you very well at the mountain peak."

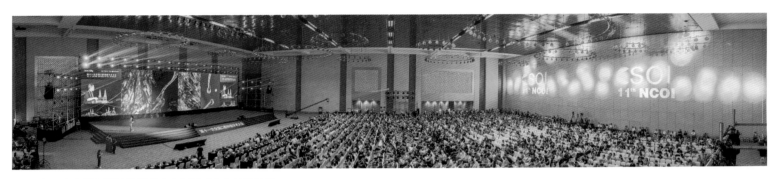

2019 年，在全国口腔种植学术大会开幕式上作特邀演讲

In 2019, an invited speech at the opening of National Conference on Oral Implantology

在同为"口腔病理学家"和"摄影师"的李铁军身上，我们看到了"科学"与"艺术"的水乳交融、相得益彰，这正是李铁军的艺术探索带给我们的财富。

In Li Tiejun, who is an "oral pathologist" as well as a "photographer", we have seen that "science" and "art" are in harmony and complement each other. This is the wealth that Li Tiejun's artistic exploration brings us.

文字转载自《北医人》2014 年第 2 期

The text of this article is reproduced from " Periodical - *The Beiyiren* ", Issue 2, 2014

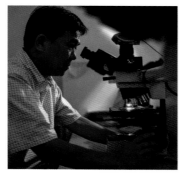
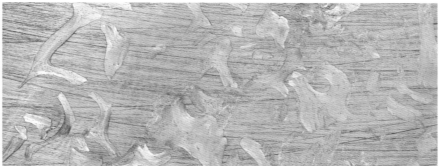

李铁军

1979—1984 年，武汉大学口腔医学院本科。

1984—1987 年，武汉大学口腔医学院硕士。

1992—1995 年，英国伯明翰大学牙学院博士。

1995—1998 年，日本鹿儿岛大学齿学部博士后。

现任北京大学口腔医学院副院长，口腔病理科主任，教授、博士生导师。兼任中华口腔医学会常务理事、中华口腔医学会口腔生物医学专业委员会主任委员、中华口腔医学会口腔病理学专业委员会副主任委员等职。

主要研究方向为颌骨牙源性囊肿和肿瘤的生长特征与临床行为。2006 年获国家杰出青年科学基金资助，曾获国家 863 子课题、国家自然科学基金重点项目资助。

迄今在国内外发表学术论文 100 余篇，其中 SCI 收录 78 篇；2014—2018 年爱思唯尔 Scopus 数据库发布的中国高被引学者榜单上，连续 5 年被列在医学类前 100 位学者；主编专著 7 部。

2001 年获中国高校自然科学奖二等奖，2005 年获教育部提名国家科学技术奖自然科学奖二等奖，2006 年获北京市科技进步奖三等奖。

享受国务院政府特殊津贴待遇，2011 年获"卫生部有突出贡献中青年专家"称号，2012 年获中国科协"全国优秀科技工作者"称号。

李铁军教授业余爱好摄影，中国摄影家协会会员。曾出版《生命之美》显微摄影写意集，在国内外大学和艺术博物馆举办数次个人影展，其显微摄影作品在多种摄影专业期刊和媒体上发表。

Dr. Li Tiejun

Dr. Li Tiejun graduated from Wuhan University School of Stomatology in 1984, and later obtained his PhD in the University of Birmingham Dental School (UK) in 1995. He then worked as a postdoctoral fellow in Kagoshima University Dental School (Japan) during 1995-1998.

At present, he is the vice dean of Peking University School of Stomatology, professor in oral pathology. He has a long-standing research interest in the growth and behavior of odontogenic lesions of the jaws. He has won a number of academic awards throughout his career and has also been the recipient of numerous research grants from various resources.

Most notably, he has been awarded National Science Fund for Distinguished Young Scholars in 2006 by the Chinese National Natural Science Foundation. To date, he has published over 100 scientific papers, and has also been the editor to 6 monographs and major contributor to 8 other books.

Professor Li is a photography amateur, a member of China Photography Association. He has published an album of photomicrographs illustrating the beauty of life. Several art exhibitions of his photomicrographs have been held in universities of home and abroad as well as in the art museums. His art works have been widely distributed in professional photography journals and media in China.

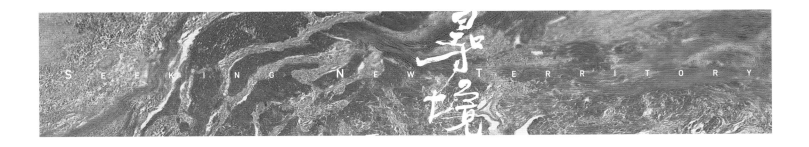

图书在版编目（CIP）数据

寻境：生命之美显微摄影艺术 / 李铁军著 . 一北
京：人民卫生出版社，2021.7
ISBN 978-7-117-31765-8

I. ①寻…　II. ①李…　III. ①显微摄影 - 医学摄影 -
摄影集　IV. ①R445-64

中国版本图书馆 CIP 数据核字（2021）第 116086 号

| 人卫智网 | www.ipmph.com | 医学教育、学术、考试、健康，
购书智慧智能综合服务平台 |
| 人卫官网 | www.pmph.com | 人卫官方资讯发布平台 |

策划编辑　鲁志强　白晓旭
责任编辑　鲁志强　白晓旭
书籍设计　正视文化
责任设计　郭　淼
书名题字　王延鹏

寻境——生命之美显微摄影艺术
Xunjing——Shengming Zhi Mei Xianwei Sheying Yishu

著　　者　李铁军
出版发行　人民卫生出版社（中继线 010-59780011）
地　　址　北京市朝阳区潘家园南里 19 号
邮　　编　100021
E - mail　pmph @ pmph.com
购书热线　010-59787592　010-59787584　010-65264830
印　　刷　北京顶佳世纪印刷有限公司
经　　销　新华书店
开　　本　889×1194　　1/12
印　　张　15.5
字　　数　312 千字
版　　次　2021 年 7 月第 1 版
印　　次　2021 年 8 月第 1 次印刷
标准书号　ISBN 978-7-117-31765-8
定　　价　228.00 元

打击盗版举报电话：010-59787491　E-mail：WQ @ pmph.com
质量问题联系电话：010-59787234　E-mail：zhiliang @ pmph.com